MW00630444

Sauna Therapy

For

Detoxification and Healing

Dr. Lawrence Wilson

Copyright © 2003, 2006, 2011, 2014, 2016, 2017

L.D. Wilson Consultants, Inc.
P.O. Box 54
Prescott, AZ 86302-0054

All rights reserved

ISBN   0-9628657-6-1

Other books by Dr. Wilson:

Nutritional Balancing and Hair Mineral Analysis
Legal Guidelines for Unlicensed Practitioners
The Real Self

To order books, please visit www.drlwilson.com or www.Amazon.com

Warning and Disclaimer. Information and any instructions provided are not intended as diagnosis, treatment or prescription for any disease or condition. Always seek professional guidance for any health condition before undertaking a sauna therapy program. One can die in a sauna due to electrolyte imbalances, accidents or improper use of the sauna. However, sauna therapy is quite safe when conducted responsibly.

Table of Contents

1. INTRODUCTION TO SAUNAS 1
Sauna History 2
Five Ways To Use Saunas 2
Eliminating Organic Chemicals 3
Removing Toxic Metals 3
Clearing Biological Toxins...................... 5
Eliminating Ionizing Radiation 6
An Anti-aging Therapy............................ 7
Practical Considerations 7

2. THE EFFECTS OF SAUNAS 9
The Two Phases Of A Sauna Session...... 9

Effects Common To All Saunas 10
Phase One Effects For All Saunas 10
Phase Two Effects For All Saunas 13
Other Effects Of Far Infrared Saunas 15
Other Effects Of Infrared Lamp Saunas 16
Effects On Body Organs And Systems . 18
Effects Of Saunas On the Oxidation Rate
.... 19
Saunas And Weight Loss....................... 19
Do Saunas Burn Calories? 20
Adding Energy To The Body 20
Heating The Acupuncture Meridians 20

Comparison Of Sauna Effects With Those of
Related Therapies 21
Fever Therapies, Hot Baths, Hot Tubs
And Steam Baths Versus Saunas........... 21
Electric Blankets Versus Saunas 21
Exercise Versus Saunas 22
Fasting Versus Saunas 22

3. HEAT SHOCK PROTEINS 23
Renaturation 24
Heat Shock Therapy 24
Analogous Concepts 25
Other Metabolic Effects 25
HSPs And Nutrition................................ 25
Coley's Toxins And HSPs 26
Sauna Protocol And HSPs 26

4. SAUNA PROTOCOL 27
Types Of Saunas Used For Therapy 27
Traditional Saunas 27
Far Infrared Saunas................................ 28
Infrared Lamp Saunas............................ 28
Enclosures Versus Cabinets 29
Cost And Outfitting. 30
Steam 30
When To Use A Sauna 30
How Often To Use A Sauna 31
How Long To Remain In A Sauna 31
Sauna Danger Signals 32
How Much Sauna Therapy 32
Replenishing Minerals 32
Before A Sauna Session 33
During And After A Sauna Session....... 34
Supervision 35
Relaxation... 35
Sauna Therapy During Acute Infections 36
Cautions And Contraindications............ 36

5. DETOXIFICATION........................ 41
The Philosophy Of Detoxification......... 41
Sauna Detoxification Mechanisms 42
Heating The Body.................................. 42
Skin Activation 42
Sweating 43
Hot And Dry (Yang) Effects 43
Improving Circulation 44
Strengthening The Parasympathetic
Nervous System..................................... 44
Relieving Internal Congestion 45
Normalizing Alkalinity.......................... 45
Enhancing Oxygenation 45
Deep Tissue Penetration 45
Other Infrared Benefits 45
Seven Approaches To Eliminate Toxins 45
Other Detoxification Topics 48
Preferred Minerals 48
Layered Toxins 49
To Detoxify, Remove The Need For
Compensations 49
Order Of Organ Cleanout 50

Toxins Versus Genetics 50
The Concept Of Density 50
Healing Facility Or Home Therapy 51
Home-based Therapy 51
Potential Detoxification Program
    Difficulties 51

6. OTHER ASPECTS OF SAUNA THERAPY 53
Visualization 53
Aromatherapy 54
Sound 54
Conscious Breathing 54
Posture 55
Eye Exercises 56
Color 56
Exercise 57
Reflexology And Massage 57
Water 57
Steam 57
Ozone 58
Niacin 58
Cool Bathing And Cold Plunges 58
Charcoal Tablets 59
Vitamin D 59

7. A MORE COMPLETE HEALING PROGRAM 61
Diet 61
Beverages 64
Supplementary Nutrients 65
Rest 65
Exercise 66
Healing Attitudes 66
Healthful Relationships 66
Other Natural Therapies 67
Clothing, Breathing And Thoughts 67
Medications 68

8. EFFECTS ON HEALTH CONDITIONS 69
Cardiovascular System 69
Multiple Chemical Sensitivity Or MCS 70
Drug Detoxification 70

Pesticide, Chemical And Toxic Metal
Exposure 71
Nervous System Disorders 71
Musculo-skeletal Conditions 72
Skin Conditions 72
Ear, Nose and Throat Conditions 72
Eye Conditions 73
Digestive Disorders 73
Reproductive Conditions 73
Other 73

9. SAUNAS AND INFECTIOUS DISEASE 75
Heating The Body 75
Improving Circulation 76
Improved Oxygenation 76
Sweating 76
Effects Of Infrared Radiation 76
Deep Heat Penetration 76
Sympathetic Nervous System Inhibition 77
Production Of Heat Shock Proteins 77
Enhancing Digestion 77
Light And Color Therapy 77
No Side Effects Or Tolerance 78
Combining With Other Therapies 78
Inexpensive And Available To All 78
Sauna Use In Acute Infections 78
Saunas Use For Chronic Infections 79
Epidemics And Pandemics 80

10. SAUNAS AND CANCER 81
What Is Cancer? 81
Estrogen, A Primary Carcinogen 82
Reduced Pancreatic Enzyme Secretion . 84
Role Of The Autonomic Nervous System
.... 84
Sauna Mechanisms For Cancer 85
Saunas and the Mental State 87
Tumor Necrosis, Pain Control, Ascites . 87
Other Therapy Considerations 87

11. HEALING REACTIONS 89
Why Healing Reactions Occur 89
Symptoms Of Healing Reactions 90

Distinguishing Healing From Disease
Reactions 91
Emotional Reactions 91
Handling Physical Healing Reactions ... 93
Specific Supportive Measures 94
Discussing Healing Reactions 96

12. SAUNA DESIGN 97
Heat Sources 97
Convection Saunas 97
Radiant Heating 98
Two Types Of Infrared Saunas 98
Hot Sand Or Solar Power 99
Electromagnetic Fields 99

Cabinets and Enclosures 99
Materials 100
Insulation 100
Size 100
Sitting, Lying Or Standing Up 101
Shape 101
Portability 102
Thermometers 102
Thermostats 102
Timers 102
Ventilation 103
Inability To Heat Up 103
Rotting 103

13. LAMP SAUNA CONSIDERATIONS
.... 105
Lying Down Or Sitting 105
For Those Who Are Bedridden 106
Cautions Regarding Aiming A Lamp
Directly At The Head 107
Lamps To Warm The Legs 107
Guards For Lamps 108
Multiple-Person Lamp saunas 108
Why Lamps On Only One Wall? 108
Converting A Sauna 109
Other Design Considerations 109
Bathroom And Closet Installation 111
Lamp Safety 112
Lamp Breakage 112
Dimmer Switches 113
Looking At Reddish Infrared Lamps ... 113

Rotating The Body During A Session 113
Other Lamp Sauna Considerations 114

14. PERSONAL EXPERIENCE WITH
AN INFRARED LAMP SAUNA 117
Sauna Protocol 117
Healing Reactions 118
Validation 120

15. SAUNA RESEARCH 125
Research Protocols 125
Sauna Therapy Program Features 126

16. REVIEW AND CONCLUSION 129
Toxic Metals And Toxic Chemicals 129
Infrared 129
Saunas And Detoxification 130
Chronic Infections 130
Other Health Conditions 130
Spiritual Renewal 130
Other Modalities Combined 130
Conclusion 131

**Appendix A. Saunas And Hair Mineral
Analysis 133**

**Appendix B. Restoring The Sympathetic
Nervous System 137**

**Appendix C. Notes For Practitioners .. 141
Sauna Disclaimer Statement 141**

**Appendix D. Infrared Sauna Electrical
Unit Plans 142**

**Appendix E. PVC Pipe Frame Enclosure
Construction Plans 146**

**Appendix F. Benefits of An Isolated
Infrared Lamp 149**

**Appendix G. Differences between the
types of saunas 151
Glossary 151
Resources 156
References 157
Index 165**

Preface

Thirty-seven years ago my brother's cancer diagnosis led me to investigate natural methods of healing. I read about the Hunza people who were cancer-free, perhaps due to their diet and lifestyle. At the time, I was an undergraduate at the Massachusetts Institute of Technology. Their Department of Nutrition gave me a grant to study the relationship between diet and cancer.

I spent weeks reading on the subject at the Harvard Medical School Library and later at the New York Academy of Medicine Library. I read the work of Max Gerson, MD, William Frederich Koch, MD Weston Price, DDS, Melvin Page, DDS and others. I also studied Macrobiotics with Michio Kushi, raw foods with Ann Wigmore and iridology with Dr. Bernard Jensen. After graduating from college, I went to medical school and while a student worked as medical director at a Natural Hygiene fasting spa. I learned much about total biological healing from all these teachers.

On graduating from medical school, I began a family practice residency at the University of Cincinnati Medical Center, but left early and for this reason never obtained a medical license. My own health had deteriorated and today I would have been diagnosed with chronic fatigue syndrome. I moved to Phoenix, Arizona to restore my health. There a friend started me on the Kelley metabolic cancer protocol. Dr. William Kelley recovered from pancreatic cancer utilizing a healing program that involved metabolic typing, coffee enemas and many nutritional supplements. This helped me get back on my feet and gave me an opportunity to experience a comprehensive metabolic healing program.

Within a year I took over the friend's nutrition consulting practice and soon met Dr. Paul C. Eck. He used hair analysis for nutritional assessment and offered to teach it to me. I had tried hair analysis before. After speaking with several laboratories, I had decided they did not understand it and it was probably a fad.

Dr. Eck uniquely interpreted hair analysis using general systems theory along with metabolic typing, the stages of stress and oxidation rates, concepts which others were not using. I began to incorporate his ideas on myself and with patients, with excellent results. I set about learning it and worked with Dr. Eck one day a week for over 10 years. I wrote about his marvelous work in *Nutritional Balancing and Hair Mineral Analysis*.

In 1996, I moved to cleaner surroundings in Prescott, Arizona. Although aware of sauna therapy, I had little idea of its benefits or how to use saunas properly. After all, how could such a simple therapy be so effective? I would soon learn about the power of the *combination* of heat, color, sympathetic nervous system inhibition, increased circulation and infrared energy.

In early 2002, a friend suggested experimenting with infrared lamps to heat up a sauna. Though not readily available commercially, John Harvey Kellogg, MD had recommended lamp saunas over 100 years ago. I converted an old hot air sauna to a lamp sauna and began an intense therapy program. Chapter 14 describes the dramatic results, including the changes in my hair tissue mineral analyses. I began recommending sauna therapy to clients, observing excellent results.

In this age of toxic exposure and drug-resistant infections, saunas are indeed a great blessing. Combined with a complete healing program, no other single technique has so impressed me. Unable to find books about sauna therapy, I decided to write one. This volume documents the protocols, rationales and research I have found so far about the use of this ancient, safe, inexpensive and very potent natural healing method.

Many, many people contributed to this book. I cannot recall all the doctors, clients and friends who asked hard questions that led me to experiment and research more deeply. In particular, many thanks to my friend, R.W., for the idea of using infrared heat lamps in a sauna. For editing, many thanks to Megan Lorimer. The cover design is by Beverly Allisone. Cartoons are by Monica Mueller.

Lawrence Wilson
April 2006

Preface To The 2011 Edition

This edition is similar to the older one. I added small sections about meditation, colon cleansing, and coffee enemas and corrected several small errors about the general diet and drinking water. Further updates will be found at **www.drlwilson.com.** Feedback from several hundred people who have either built or purchased near infrared light saunas continues to indicate that:

1. Sauna therapy is safe, powerful, and quite comfortable for most people. It can be a truly remarkable addition to any healing regimen. It continues to be an amazing and very important aspect of nutritional balancing science.

2. I would avoid the type of sauna that claims to be adjustable for either near or far infrared. It is not nearly the same as a red heat lamp sauna.

3. The near infrared light sauna appears to be the best type of sauna for detoxification. The other types of saunas such as a traditional hot rocks sauna or the far infrared type will work to some degree, but are not as effective because:

a) These operate at higher temperatures so they are less comfortable for some people.

b) They do not penetrate the skin as deeply, and they cannot be used for 'spot therapy' because the heat is distributed too evenly.

c) They do not put out the same frequencies as a NIR sauna, and they do not include the reddish color therapy.

d) Far infrared saunas, if genuine, always seems to emit some harmful electromagnetic fields that detract from their benefits.

Preface To The 2014 Edition

This edition is very similar to the earlier ones, except I have updated the diet section and about ten pages of other additions and corrections.

1
Introduction to Saunas

"I was exposed to the chemical toxins in New York City on 9/11. Ever since, 1 have had respiratory problems. My immune system took a terrible hit. I became susceptible to every cold and flu, and had bronchitis for three winters.

I have been using an infrared lamp sauna for eight months and have found it extraordinarily helpful. It has made an enormous difference. It has changed my life. The bronchitis is gone. When I get a cold I do the infrared and seem to be responding better and better. I no longer have sinus infections and the chest seems to heal with the infrared sauna.

I am also losing weight and just feeling better all around. My teeth and gums have improved, as I always had gum disease and was worried about this. In the sauna, I become centered. It is the most relaxing experience I have ever encountered, and I have done many natural therapies. I am amazed at what the sauna has done for my life already." - Mrs. D.R, Kunkletown, PA.

Sauna, a Scandinavian word, is an ancient form of heat therapy that is used in many cultures around the world. The word sauna refers to *dry* heat, although steam may be added in traditional saunas, usually by sprinkling water on hot rocks.

A sauna has two components, a *heat source* and an *enclosure* to contain the heat. The heat source may be a wood, gas or electric furnace, hot rocks, far infrared emitters or electric infrared lamps.

Enclosures can encompass the entire body such as a sweat lodge or a sauna room. Also available are sauna cabinets, where one's head remains outside.

The basic idea of a sauna is to heat the body several degrees. The body then attempts to reduce its temperature by driving blood to the surface and by sweating. Heating the body, and the body's response to heating cause many beneficial physiological effects. Infrared adds an additional set of benefits. Color therapy provided by infrared heat lamps in an infrared lamp sauna adds even more benefits.

Saunas dramatically improve circulation and relieve internal congestion. Heating the body helps destroy bacteria, viruses and tumors. Sweating promotes the elimination of toxic metals and chemicals, radioactive particles and other toxins. The skin's ability to eliminate poisons increases. Saunas offer many of the benefits of exercise while requiring much less exertion.

Several degrees

Sauna History

Hot baths have been used by virtually all indigenous cultures for several thousand years. Among them are the Mayan sweat lodge, the Mexican *temescal*, the Islamic *hammam*, the Russian *bania*, the Japanese *mushi-buro*, the Native American *sweat lodge*, as well as hot baths described in Indian Ayurvedic medical literature. Ancient Egyptian texts including the Edwin Smith Papyrus mention the use of heat therapy for tumors. The best-known European sauna users are the Finns. Hot air baths are also common among Greeks, Romans, Germans, Turks and others.

In traditional Finnish society, the sauna was a multipurpose building. Besides the weekly family baths, the building was used for smoking and curing meats, doing laundry, drying thatch, malting barley and drying fish nets. It was also used for massage, nursing the sick, washing the dead and as a birthing chamber.

Finnish settlers in America brought their sauna concepts with them. Often they would build the sauna first. It would serve as a temporary shelter to live in while they were building a house. Pioneers in natural therapeutics also employed the sauna as a healing modality. The best-known nineteenth century American sauna proponent was John Harvey Kellogg, M.D. At his sanitarium in Battle Creek, Michigan he carefully researched various dry and wet heat baths to assess their value as healing modalities. A favorite of his was the "electric light bath", employing the new incandescent light bulb. Dr. Kellogg recognized the penetrating power of the radiant heat given off by electric lamps. His device never caught on in America, but thousands were sold in Europe, including to members of the royal families.

Sauna use waned during the early years of the twentieth century, outshined by the technological wonders of modern medicine. Over the past thirty years, however, its use has increased, especially as a safe and powerful method of eliminating addictive drugs and environmental toxins. The infrared sauna was also introduced. It provides a more pleasant experience for many people and appears to be more effective for detoxification as well.

Five Ways To Use Saunas

This book focuses on sauna therapy. However, saunas may be used in several ways:

- *Relaxation.* The warm heat of a sauna relaxes the muscles and nervous system. Tensions melt away. The sauna offers a healthful method to unwind after a difficult day.

- *Health Maintenance.* Periodic use of a sauna, once a week or so, enhances circulation which nourishes the glands, cleanses the skin and offers many of the benefits of exercise.

- *Social Interaction.* Baths, saunas and sweat lodges can be community gathering places for families and other groups. The warmth promotes openness and a community spirit.

- *Spiritual Development.* Native Americans and other groups use sweat lodges for sacred ceremonies. The warmth, atmosphere and shape of the lodge make it excellent for emotional and spiritual reflection. Together with others or alone, the sauna is a marvelous place to contemplate, meditate, pray and release fears and negativity. Adding sound, color, aromatherapy and other modalities can enhance the effects of the heat.

- *Healing.* Spending from 30 minutes up to several hours per day in a sauna is a powerful yet very safe healing modality. The sauna is excellent to add fiery yang energy to the body, decongest the internal organs, assist circulation, heal infections and can help many other body systems as well.

    Standard medical therapies too often focus on relieving symptoms, while ignoring deeper causes that the sauna addresses. Among these, one of the most important is the role of toxic substances in causing ill health.

    Removing chemical, metal, biological and radioactive toxins from the body is a prime rationale for the use of saunas by everyone at this time in history. The following sections summarize the major toxins we must cope with, as well as a few conditions the sauna can help ameliorate.

Eliminating Organic Chemicals

Never before in history have large numbers of people been exposed to such a great variety and high levels of toxic chemicals. From building materials and home furnishings to food additives, solvents and thousands of other products, chemicals are part of the modern lifestyle. I will only summarize some of the classes of harmful chemicals, as many books cover this subject in detail. Common toxic chemicals include formaldehyde, phenols, xenobiotics (pesticides) and phthalates. Others include PCBs, trichloroethylene and volatile organic compounds (VOCs) found in hundreds of common products.

Often, the effects of these chemicals are subtle and cumulative. They accumulate in the water and the air, so no location remains unaffected. Avoiding exposure is all but impossible. According to the United States Environmental Protection Agency (EPA), toxic chemicals are the worst environmental problem in the nation, responsible for up to 80% of cancer deaths.

One class of chemicals, pesticides and herbicides, are among the most toxic substances known to mankind. Several billion pounds are sprayed each year directly onto our crops. Besides eating and wearing the residues, they may contaminate the air and water supplies for hundreds of years.

Testing for thousands of chemicals is costly when tests even exist, and modern medicine has little to offer to eliminate them from the body. The diseases they cause have become epidemics. Sauna therapy shines brightly as a simple, effective therapeutic modality to help eliminate chemical toxins from the body.

Removing Toxic Metals

According to the United States EPA, toxic metals are the second worst environmental problem. Pesticides may contain lead, copper, arsenic and other metals. About forty million mercury amalgam dental fillings are still placed in Americans each year. Tons of mercury is dumped into the air from coal-burning power plants and paper-making. Aluminum compounds

pesticides — lead, copper, Ar^{3}, etc Pb^{8+} Cu^{2+}
herbicides
metals — Mercury Hg^{2+} Al^{+3}

are routinely added to table salt and municipal drinking water supplies. Arsenic and lead used in pesticides and insecticides find their way into the water and the food supplies.

In my experience, everyone has excess toxic metals, whether or not they show up on any test. Most often, they are hidden deep within the brain, the liver and in many other organs and tissues as well. Some toxic metals replace vital minerals in enzyme binding sites. However, the toxic metals do not function nearly as well. As they accumulate, they contribute to hundreds of physical and emotional health conditions.

Lead contributes to more than 100 conditions including neuromuscular and bone diseases, fractures, mental retardation, hyperactivity, anemia and others. Some historians believe the Roman Empire fell because lead water pipes slowly poisoned the people and decreased their strength and intelligence. Sources of lead include old paint, inks, pesticides, a few hair dyes, solder and other metal products. During sauna therapy, I have observed that lead may have a sickly sweet odor as it is eliminated. Elimination of lead was confirmed with hair mineral testing.

Cadmium contributes to high blood pressure, heart disease, cancer, fatigue, arthritis, violence, infections, back pain and other conditions. Common sources are cigarette smoke, refined foods and tap water. A person may feel very tired for a few days when cadmium is eliminated quickly from the body.

Mercury toxicity is present in almost everyone today. Mercury is found in silver amalgam dental fillings, tuna and swordfish, most products from the sea to some extent, contact lens solution, vaccines and air pollution. Mercury may contribute to hypothyroidism, an impaired immune system, digestive problems such as yeast infections, emotional difficulties, learning disabilities, autism, ADHD and many other conditions. Mercury elimination, if heavy, may be accompanied by a fishy odor during a sauna session.

Aluminum is associated with memory impairment, Alzheimer's disease and other dementias. Aluminum compounds are found in table salt, beverage cans and aluminum foils, antiperspirants, antiacids, aluminum cookware and as a drinking water additive. Peppermint, spearmint and wintergreen are naturally high in aluminum.

Fluoride contributes to brown staining of the teeth, weakened bones, hip fractures, hypothyroidism, mental impairment, birth defects and cancer. Fluoride compounds are found in pesticides, air pollution, prescription drugs such as Prozac, toothpastes, and are added to many water supplies. Foods processed with water including baby foods and juices often contain too much fluoride. Fluoride is extremely toxic and difficult to remove from tap water.

Large, worldwide studies show little or no benefit of fluoride for tooth decay, contrary to many news reports. Only the United States, Australia and Great Britain continue to add highly toxic fluoride compounds to their drinking water.

Chlorine toxicity is associated with fatigue, heart disease, cancer and kidney problems. Chloride is required in the body and is found in salt and other foods. Many chlorinated compounds, however, are highly toxic. These include chlorinated compounds in tap water such as chloramines and chlorinated hydrocarbons used in pesticides and other chemicals. Exposure sources include bathing in chlorinated water, pools and hot tubs, and the use of chlorine bleach and other chlorine-containing household products.

Arsenic contributes to liver and kidney damage, weakness, diarrhea, muscle spasms, headaches and other symptoms. Sources include pesticides, beer, tap water, table salt, paints and other chemical products.

Physiological minerals may also become toxic in certain forms. For example, hexavalent chromium is toxic while trivalent chromium is not. Vital minerals may also become toxic if the body is missing other minerals required for their proper metabolism. For example, *calcium* is needed in the bones. When it accumulates in the arteries, joints, kidneys or elsewhere it becomes toxic. This can occur because other minerals such as sodium and copper that are required for proper calcium metabolism may become deficient or biologically unavailable.

A similar situation occurs with *iron, manganese, chromium, copper, selenium* and other vital minerals, contributing to many health conditions. Of these, the most commonly seen are copper, iron and manganese toxicity. They will often be revealed on a hair mineral test at some point if one pursues a corrective nutrition and sauna therapy program. All three of these minerals can help support weak adrenal glands.

Copper is found in many foods, especially nuts, seeds, grains and beans. Zinc deficiency and adrenal exhaustion, both very common, aggravate copper toxicity. Copper imbalance can contribute to emotional conditions, skin problems, joint pain, cancer, migraine headaches and premenstrual tension. The symptoms of copper toxicity are identical to the symptoms of premenstrual tension. Copper elimination in a sauna may be accompanied by a rotten egg odor. This may be due to sulfur that is bound to copper and eliminated along with it to protect the body from the worst effects of excessive copper.

Manganese is found in unleaded gasoline and foods such as tea. Both copper and manganese are needed in the body. However, the body may accumulate excessive manganese to help support weak adrenal glands. This manganese is not helpful and must be eliminated. Manganese elimination in a sauna may cause a slightly metallic odor.

Iron toxicity is also common, although often not revealed on standard tests. Inorganic iron is added to refined white flour products such as breads, breakfast cereal, crackers and pastry. Vitamin and mineral supplements often contain iron. Iron can accumulate to help support weak adrenal glands. It is stored in the liver and other organs and may contribute to heart disease, cancer, emotional difficulties and other health problems.

Sauna therapy is excellent to remove excess minerals, both toxic metals and unusable and excessive amounts of physiological minerals.

Clearing Biological Toxins

Chronic infections play an important role in many health conditions. These range from artery disease and ulcers to arthritis and perhaps some cancers. Many bacteria and fungi in particular produce powerful toxins that contribute to both local and systemic disease. Endotoxins are those produced within bacteria that often cause fevers and many other symptoms. Exotoxins are those secreted by bacteria. According to *Dorland's Illustrated Medical Dictionary*, they are among the most poisonous substances known to mankind.

5

Endotoxins — produced w/in bacteria
Exotoxins — secreted by bacteria

Weakened by exposure to toxic chemicals and heavy metals, the bodies today are much more susceptible to attack by infections. More and more infections are becoming resistant to drug therapy as a result of weakened bodies and the overuse of antibiotics.

Viral infections such as AIDS, Hanta and West Nile virus, Avian flu and many, many others are also on the rise and difficult to treat conventionally. Other infections difficult to treat with conventional means such as Lyme disease are also increasing in frequency. Many infections today are chronic, causing nagging complaints that never go away. This occurs especially in areas of the body with poor circulation such as the joints, ears and sinuses.

Heating the body is a natural mechanism the body uses to fight infections. Indeed, a low body temperature due to impaired thyroid activity or other factors is one of the causes of recurrent infections. Sauna therapy not only heats the body, but powerfully improves circulation and employs other mechanisms as well to help fight both acute and chronic infections. This topic is discussed in detail in Chapter 9.

Eliminating Ionizing Radiation

An article in *The Ecologist*, April 2001 issue, begins by stating, "the (radiation) equivalent of a nuclear war has already happened". This may not be an exaggeration. The article carefully details that 1900 nuclear tests, accidents and nuclear waste dumping have exposed everyone on the planet to the equivalent of 100 Hiroshima bombs.

The article reveals details of previously classified accidents, including one in Greenland in 1968. A B-52 crashed at a secret nuclear base and its cargo of four nuclear bombs detonated, sending up a cloud of plutonium 25,000 feet into the air. According to US documents, 1250 nuclear weapons have been involved in accidents, a number of which "resulted in or created the potential for plutonium dispersal". The Soviet Union was notorious for its cavalier attitude regarding nuclear accidents. A 1991 film documents the poisoning of hundreds of thousands as a result of accidents at their first plutonium factory at Chelyabinsk in the Ural Mountains.

Using the official 'radiation risk' estimates published in 1991 by the International Commission on Radiological Protection, planetwide contamination will cause 175 million cancer deaths and another 350 million non-fatal cancers. It will also cause another 235 million illnesses and 588 million children to be born with birth defects such as brain damage, mental disability, spina bifida and others.

Depleted uranium, a waste product which every nation that has atomic weapons has in abundance, is another source of radiation exposure. To get rid of it, it is often made into ammunition that was used in the Gulf War, Bosnia and Kosovo. Leukemia rates have increased in these areas since its use.

Another hidden source of radiation is the fluoride compounds added to many municipal water supplies. Hydrofluosilicic acid, the source of most fluoride for water supplies, is a smokestack waste product that contains radioactive particles along with the fluoride.

Other sources are medical and dental x-rays, medical waste that may contain radioactive materials, CAT and other scans, smoke alarms and proximity to food irradiation facilities.

Radiation is carried on mineral particles. The minerals lodge in the cells where they disrupt DNA synthesis. This causes defective protein synthesis resulting in innumerable subtle metabolic dysfunctions. As the defective proteins replicate, the metabolic errors also multiply.

Kids *x1/week*

Infrared lamp sauna therapy promotes more rapid turnover of damaged body cells. The deeply penetrating energy helps kill damaged cells, which are often more heat-sensitive than normal cells. Eliminating the radiation-containing cells helps the body eliminate radioactive particles faster and prevents replication of these cells. Over a period of time, lamp sauna therapy can thus reduce the amount of mutated DNA and radioactive material in the body. One needs to continue sauna use on a maintenance basis because exposure to radiation continues throughout one's life.

An Anti-aging Therapy

As we age, a number of changes take place that are reversed to varying degrees with sauna therapy. These include a slower metabolic rate, less sweating, slower healing and a reduced ability to eliminate toxins and infections. These changes contribute to the risk of major illness and to the process of aging. Since sauna therapy helps reverse them, it may be considered a prime anti-aging therapy.

Sauna therapy can be of tremendous value for a wide variety of conditions. It can be used by most people at any age, even by those in wheelchairs. Physicians familiar with it contend that it can be adapted for any condition with proper supervision. Simple yet powerful, it can usually be done right in the home.

Practical Considerations

The FDA approves of saunas as therapeutic devices. Consult with your health insurance representative regarding reimbursement for the cost of a sauna. The Internal Revenue Service may consider sauna therapy a deductible health expense if prescribed by a doctor.

Adding a built-in sauna will increase the value of one's home. Unlike hot tubs and steam rooms, saunas require practically no maintenance and are simple and inexpensive to operate.

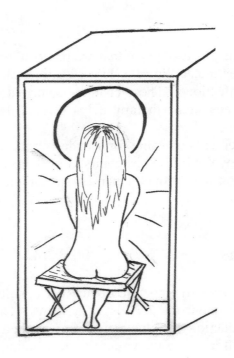

"Women don't sweat!   They glow."

2
The Effects of Saunas

"It is incredible! In just a few short weeks of using an infrared lamp sauna, I am beginning to feel so much better. I have seen so many physicians and spent so much money with no results. It is wonderful to be free of amitrytiline (an anti-depressant drug), and my hopes for the future are looking brighter. I have finally found something that really helps."
- Mrs. D.A., Phoenix, Arizona.

The great benefits of saunas are due to *a combination of a dozen or more physiological effects*. This is the wonderful secret of the healing power of the sauna. In this chapter, sauna benefits are divided into those that occur early in a sauna session and those that occur later in the session. These two phases of a sauna session I have called *Phase One* and *Phase Two*.

The Two Phases of a Sauna Session

The effects of saunas occur in two phases. The distinction is important for sauna therapy. In the *first phase*, the body temperature remains approximately at basal level and sweating is light. Although tissue heating occurs, the body is able to dissipate the extra heat by increasing circulation, shunting blood to the skin and sweating. As a result, the body temperature does not rise.

Phase one sauna effects include inhibiting the sympathetic nervous system, inducing sweating, relieving pain, reducing heat production, improving oxygenation and dilating peripheral blood vessels. Others are relieving internal organ congestion, relaxing the muscles and enhancing the flexibility of tendons and ligaments.

Phase Two. After 10 to 30 minutes, the body can no longer dissipate the heat of the sauna. Body temperature rises. Blood is more forcefully shunted to the surface. The heart rate and sweating increase. One may feel feverish with slightly labored breathing and some faintness or light-headedness. It may be tempting to get out of the sauna, but this is not recommended unless discomfort is extreme. Some of the greatest benefits occur during the second phase of a session.

Phase two sauna effects include increasing the body temperature and hastening the death of weaker cells. They also include further increasing the heart rate and circulation. Others are directly disabling pathogenic microorganisms, resolving infiltrates and exudates and normalizing enzymatic activity when basal body temperature is low. Some researchers believe infrared sauna therapy also produces heat shock proteins.

When starting sauna therapy, the second phase may begin in 10 minutes. As one acclimates to the sauna over several weeks to months, phase two may occur somewhat later in a session. Body temperature often rises abruptly in the second phase. One can check this by taking one's temperature every few minutes during a sauna session. It will often remain at basal level and then suddenly rise a few degrees. The body may be resetting its thermostat to a higher temperature, as occurs in infectious illnesses.

After a sauna session, body temperature may remain elevated for up to 15 minutes or so. Then it may suddenly drop back to the basal level. One will often feel fatigued or light-headed for 10-15 minutes after a sauna session, in part for this reason. Resting ten to fifteen minutes after a sauna session is important as it gives the body a better opportunity to restore normal functioning.

Effects Common To All Saunas

Effects are described first for *all saunas*. This is followed by a discussion of effects that are unique to *infrared lamp and far infrared saunas*, and then effects unique to *infrared lamp saunas*.

Phase One Effects for all Saunas

1) Balancing The Autonomic Nervous System

Sauna therapy inhibits excessive sympathetic nervous system activity. This enhances parasympathetic activity that is required for healing. The mechanisms involved are 1) sweating, 2) enhancing peripheral circulation and 3) inhibiting normal heat production. These autonomic effects are explained below.

Balancing the autonomic nervous system is one of the most important benefits of sauna therapy. This topic is so important that a more complete explanation of the autonomic nervous system is included in Appendix B.

Many people have chronically overstimulated sympathetic nervous systems. This causes a wide range of difficulties, from adrenal exhaustion and fatigue to blood sugar problems, anxiety, poor circulation, an impaired immune system, poor digestion and impaired elimination.

Reducing excessive sympathetic nervous system activity assists the parasympathetic nervous system. This enhances immune system activity and relaxes the muscles and the nervous system. It also rests the thyroid and adrenal glands and promotes improved digestion and absorption of nutrients.

Strengthening the parasympathetic system also helps relieve blood stagnation. Chronic sympathetic stimulation due to stress forces more blood into the internal organs as part of the fight-or-flight response. Blood stagnates there, impairing the circulation and nutrition of the organs and decreasing their ability to eliminate wastes. Saunas help relieve this common cause of ill health.

2) Inducing Sweating

Evaporation of water on the skin's surface has a cooling effect. The source of the fluid in sweat is interstitial fluid. It is similar to lymph and contains many minerals and other chemicals. Any chemical in the blood or lymph may find its way into sweat.

Sweating occurs with both sympathetic and parasympathetic activity. However, it is primarily a parasympathetic activity.

> "Fibers to most sweat glands are cholinergic...the sweat glands are stimulated primarily by centers in the hypothalamus that are usually considered to be parasympathetic centers. Therefore, sweating could be called a parasympathetic function." (Guyton, p. 715)

Sweating During Exercise Versus Sweating In Saunas. Sweat generated by exercise has a different composition and is less effective for detoxification. Sympathetic activation by exercise reduces the activity of the organs of elimination and shunts blood away from these organs. Guyton's *Textbook of Medical Physiology* explains this as follows:

- "In heavy exercise, sympathetic stimulation is an absolute essential. Sympathetic stimulation has multiple effects on the circulation that are critical in increasing the cardiac output to the very high levels required in heavy exercise." (p. 279)
- "At least three different mechanisms enhance sympathetic activity during exercise." (p. 279)
- "Mass sympathetic discharge in many different ways increases the capability of the body to perform vigorous muscle activity." (p. 719)
- "Sympathetic stimulation reduces kidney output." (p. 715)

Acclimatization of the Sweating Mechanism. When beginning a sauna program, congestion and inactivity of the skin impair sweating. After weeks or perhaps up to six months of repeated sauna use, the skin becomes more active and sweating increases up to fourfold.

Acclimatization causes decreased concentration of sodium chloride in the sweat, which allows progressively better conservation of minerals. Most of this effect is caused by increased secretion of aldosterone.

> "An unacclimatized person who sweats profusely often loses as much as 15 to 30 grams of salt each day for the first few days. But, after four to six weeks of acclimatization, the loss may be as little as 3-5 grams per day." (Guyton, p. 890)

Sweating in Different Areas of the Body. When one begins a sauna program, sweating may only occur in some areas of the body. As the program progresses, more of the skin sweats.

Sweating in Men Versus Women. Men generally sweat more easily than women because men in general have faster metabolic rates that generate more heat naturally. Women usually require more time in a sauna in order to begin sweating.

3) Improving Oxygenation

Sauna therapy improves oxygenation in four ways:
- As the body attempts to reduce its temperature, more blood flows to the lungs and the skin where the blood picks up more oxygen.
- Increased pulse and stroke volume pumps more blood through the entire body.
- Repeated sauna use activates the skin, increasing its ability to transfer oxygen to the blood.
- Clearing bronchial and lung infections and congestion may also increase oxygenation.

4) Dilating Peripheral Vessels

Shunting the blood toward the body surface by dilating the peripheral blood vessels is the primary mechanism used to reduce body temperature.

> "This is caused by inhibition of the sympathetic centers in the posterior hypothalamus that cause vasoconstriction. Full vasodilation can increase the rate of heat transfer to the skin as much as 8-fold." (Guyton, p. 891)

5) Relieving Internal Congestion

In his text, *Light Therapeutics,* J.H. Kellogg, MD wrote, "passive congestion or stagnation of the blood in a (vital organ) necessarily involves diminished oxygenation and accumulation of CO2 and other toxic substances in the tissues."

Saunas powerfully move blood throughout the body. Sympathetic inhibition combined with peripheral vasodilation forces blood to the body surface, reducing congestion in the liver, kidneys and other internal organs. Dr. Kellogg noted that:

> "blood vessels of every important internal organ are very directly connected with the vessels of the skin....we possess in artificial congestion of the skin (using the sauna) a method whereby we may quickly withdraw from the great vascular organs of the trunk from one-fourth to one-half of their total contents (of blood)."

The infrared lamp sauna design suggested in this book involves rotating the body every few minutes, applying heat alternately to one side of the body and then to another. This is even more effective to relieve internal congestion than uniform heating that occurs in other types of saunas.

6) Relaxing Muscles and Enhancing Flexibility of Tendons and Ligaments

Reduced sympathetic stimulation, improved blood flow and a release of toxins all contribute to these effects.

7) Reducing Heat Production

Adding heat from an external source tends to decrease internal heat production.

"When body temperature elevates, heat production by shivering and chemical thermogenesis is strongly inhibited". (Guyton, p. 892)

Chemical thermogenesis means the biochemical generation of heat within the body. It is enhanced by greater activity of the sympathetic nervous system.

8. Increasing The Alkalinity of the System

Dr. Kellogg also knew that sweating can have a beneficial effect of normalizing the acid-alkaline balance in the body. This is determined in great part by the balance of the minerals in the body. However, toxins generally acidify the system by impairing circulation and the elimination of acid end-products of metabolism. Many bacteria and viruses also secrete acidic products that help to acidify the body.

Phase Two Effects for all Saunas:

1) Increasing Body Temperature

Raising body temperature is a basic physiological effect of saunas. Body temperature may increase 1- 4° F. Hyperthermia has the following effects:

2) Hastening The Death of Weaker Cells

Heating the tissues a few degrees for at least 15 minutes can destroy or disable weak, heat-sensitive cells. These may include:

- cancer cells.
- bacteria and spirochetes such as Borrelia burgdorferi which causes Lyme disease
- fungi and other parasites
- cells infected with viruses
- cells with damaged DNA
- cells containing radioactive minerals
- cells filled with chemical toxins
- cells containing toxic levels of metals
- other defective cells

Dr. Jeffrey Freeman, founder of the Europa Institute of Integrated Medicine, wrote that:

"Researchers have found that the blood vessels in normal tissue ... open up (dilate) when heat is applied in an effort to flush out the heat...A tumor is a more tightly packed group of cells (and) blood circulation is sluggish and restricted. When heat is applied to the tumor (circulation is inadequate and) the temperature continues to rise to destructive levels."

3) Producing Heat Shock Proteins

Recent research indicates that heating the body can temporarily suspend the synthesis of normal body proteins and instead induce production of special proteins that preserve and restore normal cell activity. These heat shock proteins (HSPs) powerfully enhance the immune system and improve cellular energy production, respiration, elimination and other cell functions.

HSPs can inhibit the growth of cancer and improve conditions such as congestive heart failure and recovery from heart attacks. Chapter 3 focuses on HSPs and their possible relation to sauna therapy.

4) Improving Genetics

Today, many people have a significant amount of damaged DNA due to the effects of toxic chemicals and ionizing radiation. Saunas assist in improving DNA three ways:

- Improving the circulation and assisting the eliminative organs helps remove radioactive particles and toxic chemicals.
- Heat shock proteins produced in sauna sessions may increase the rate of DNA replication, transcription and translation.
- Heating the body helps kill weaker mutated cells, preventing their reproduction and slowly improving the ratio of healthy cells to genetically damaged cells.

5) Increasing The Heart Rate and Enhancing Circulation

A more rapid pulse may occur and if so, it is due to increased body temperature rather than to sympathetic nervous stimulation as occurs with exercise.

"Increased temperature causes greatly increased heart rate...These effects presumably result from the heat causing increased permeability of the muscle membrane to the ions, resulting in acceleration of the self-excitation process." (Guyton, p. 162)

Increasing cardiac output while at the same time shunting blood to the body surface increases blood circulation to many areas of the body.

6) Resolving Infiltrates, Edema and Exudates

Improving circulation, disabling microorganisms and enhancing immune system activity through production of heat shock proteins can help reduce edema, infiltrates and exudates. Infiltrates are any material in a tissue that is foreign to it. Exudates are fluid, cells or cellular debris that have escaped from blood vessels and have deposited in body tissues.

7) Normalizing Enzymatic Activity When Basal Body Temperature is Low

Low basal body temperature is very common. This condition impairs the activity of thousands of enzymatic reactions, affecting every body system. Heating the body to its normal temperature temporarily corrects this condition and allows many enzymes to function better.

Effects of Far Infrared Saunas

The *far infrared sauna* is a newer type of sauna. It became available about 40 years and is heated by six to twelve ceramic or metallic heating elements. They emit radiation in a narrow far infrared frequency range.

We cannot recommend this type of sauna at all because they all emit harmful frequencies. Beware that some manufacturers are not honest about this fact. If you have a far infrared sauna, we suggest converting it to a heat lamp sauna (see page 109).

Therapeutic effects of infrared saunas may include:

1. Some Deep Tissue Heating

Far infrared radiant energy penetrates the skin and heats the tissues to about one and a half inches inside. This allows sweating to begin sooner than in hot air saunas that heat only the body surface. This also permits one to sweat at a lower ambient temperature because infrared heats the body, but not the air. Many find this a more comfortable experience and the effects are as intense or more so than those of a traditional sauna.

2. Enhancing The Activity of Water Molecules

Water molecules vibrate at infrared frequencies. Far infrared energy resonates with water molecules in the body, enhancing their energy and causing deep heating.

Resonance can produce other interesting effects on metal oxides, exciting the molecules in ways similar to the way neon and fluorescent lamps function. The addition of certain frequencies to the gases in neon tubes causes them to emit light and perhaps other frequencies.

As water moves through pipes or is processed by reverse osmosis its energy decreases. This occurs less with distillation and carbon filtration. Exposure to infrared energy helps restore activity to water molecules in the body.

3. More Yang Therapy

Chapter 5 discusses yin and yang therapies, a central concept in nutritional balancing science. Today most bodies are too yin. Consequently, yang or warming therapies are often more effective to create balance in the body. While all sauna therapy is warming, infrared heating is more yang than using the heater in a standard hot-rocks sauna.

Several Comments About Far Infrared Saunas

Claims. Sauna manufacturers and sales people may claim benefits for far infrared saunas based on studies that, in fact, were done with *infrared lamp saunas*, and not the far infrared type of sauna. One example is an article about chronic heart failure treated with saunas (Kihara, 2002). A review noted that the saunas were heated with infrared heat lamps.

Additional Effects of Infrared Lamp Saunas

Infrared lamp saunas are heated by reddish, infrared incandescent lamps, a type sold at hardware stores. Benefits of this heat source are due to full-spectrum infrared energy with most of it in the near infrared range and a little in the middle and far infrared range. Effects are also due to color therapy, more vigorous circulation due to design and other frequencies emitted by incandescent infrared lamps. These lamps can be added to almost any sauna.

1) Shortening Cluster Chains

Infrared energy shortens chains of polluted water molecules. As this occurs, pollutants such as carbon monoxide, carbon dioxide and sulfur dioxide are expelled into the air. Heavy metals such as mercury and cadmium precipitate, facilitating their removal. This is a powerful mechanism of detoxification that does not occur to the same degree in a hot air sauna or far infrared sauna.

Shortening the chains also decreases the specific gravity of the water and enhances its adherence to cell surfaces. This improves the absorption of nutrients and elimination of waste products.

2) A Tissue Nutrient

More and more evidence indicates that certain light frequencies in the red and near infrared range have very beneficial effects on the tissues. Dr. C.S. Enwemeka recently wrote regarding these benefits:

"It includes the ability to accelerate inflammation, promote fibroblast proliferation, enhance chondroplasia, upregulates the synthesis of type I and type III procollagen mRNA, quicken bone repair and remodeling, foster revascularization of wounds and overall accelerate tissue repair in experimental and clinical models." ("Therapeutic Light", *Interdis. J. of Rehab.*, Jan/Feb 2004)

3) Reducing Lipid Peroxidation and Enhancing Oxygen Production

Infrared energy reduces lipid peroxidation that takes place in all cells as a result of energy production (*Jap J of Inflammation*, 1996, 16(6)(Nov):4-5). This is helpful to preserve delicate cell structures. At the same time, it increases the production of active oxygen in neutrophils and inhibits tumor growth (*Jap J of Inflammation*, 1996, 16(6)(Nov):9).

4) Relieving Pain

Studies indicate that light therapy in the red and near infrared range can reduce pain. Studies indicate it may have direct effects on peripheral nerves and it may modulate the levels of prostaglandins in inflammatory conditions such as arthritis.

"Works from the laboratories of Drs. Shimon Rochkind of Tel-Aviv, Israel and Juanita Anders of Bethesda, MD, USA indicate that specific energy frequencies of light promote nerve regeneration, including regeneration of the spinal cord - a part of the central nervous system once considered inert to healing." ("Therapeutic Light", *Interdisc. J. Rehab.* Jan/Feb 2004)

Pain relief mechanisms may also include reducing muscle spasms and relieving ischemia due to impaired circulation. They may also include improving oxygenation of the tissues, removing irritants and toxins and disabling or killing pathogenic microorganisms.

5) Color Therapy

Color therapy is an ancient and often highly effective healing modality. The electric lamp sauna design using red infrared lamps emits red, orange and yellow light. According to traditional color concepts, the red end of the spectrum nourishes the adrenal glands, liver and kidneys. It may also act on the aura or emotional body. It also moves the chi or vital energy downward from the head toward the lower centers where it is usually deficient.

Most any sauna can be fitted with lamps to add color therapy. With the body unclothed, the sauna is a logical place to make use of this excellent healing method. More information about color is found in Chapter 6.

6) More Vigorous Circulatory Effects

In the lamp sauna design recommended in Appendix D, the lamps are all on one wall of the sauna. One must rotate the body 90° every few minutes to heat the entire body evenly. This is more effort. However, it shunts blood from one side of the body to another, vigorously enhancing the circulatory effects of the sauna.

7) Deeper Tissue Penetration and More Yang Therapy

Three powerful infrared lamps heat the tissues up to three inches inside the body, we believe. This is more than occurs with most far infrared saunas that use 6-12 less powerful elements.

8) Ability to Focus Energy

At times it is most helpful to be able to direct heat, light and infrared energy to a particular area of the body, such as a stiff back or congested sinuses. One may do this to a slight degree in a hot air or far infrared sauna by moving closer to a heat source. However, the heater in hot air saunas is recessed, making it hard to approach. The emitters or elements in a typical far infrared sauna are not powerful enough to provide much of a boost, even if one sits close to them.

The 250-watt heat lamps in an infrared lamp sauna are very intense. By moving within 12 inches of one of the lamps, one can enhance the heat, light and infrared penetration to a part of the body. One must avoid touching or splashing water on a hot lamp.

9) Enhanced Effects on DNA

The greater intensity of infrared and deeper tissue penetration of the infrared lamp sauna may increase the death or disabling of mutated cells. This assists regeneration of normal body tissue. This may be very important for those with degenerative illnesses due to damaged DNA.

Effects On Body Organs And Systems

Saunas have wide-ranging effects on many body organs and systems. This occurs because the sauna helps remove toxic metals, toxic chemicals and chronic infections. The general effect is a normalization of the functioning of the organs. Following is a summary of more specific effects based on current research. There is a great need for more research on the sauna's effects.

Kidneys. Blood is shunted away from the kidneys during sweating and directed toward the body surface. The kidneys' burden lessens during sauna use as more water and toxins are eliminated through sweating. Repeated use helps rest and restore the kidneys.

Nervous System. Sympathetic inhibition occurs during sauna use. This reduces the fight-or-flight response, strengthens the parasympathetic system and relaxes the central nervous system. Regular sauna use has a wonderfully calming effect on the nervous system.

Liver. By shunting blood to the surface, congestion of blood in the liver is reduced during sauna use. This can enhance the liver's detoxification ability. By reducing sympathetic nervous system activity, sauna use promotes bile secretion and emptying of the gall bladder.

Spleen and Pancreas. Sympathetic nervous inhibition increases pancreatic secretion of enzymes and decreases insulin and glucagon secretion. Sauna use decreases the storage of blood in the spleen, as more blood is shunted to the surface. This helps decrease congestion of the spleen.

Immune System. Sympathetic inhibition enhances some aspects of immune system activity. Heating the body several degrees can enhance white blood cell activity and disables heat-sensitive microorganisms, assisting the elimination of many infections. Heating the body in a sauna may also produce heat shock proteins that are powerful immune system stimulators.

Cardiovascular System. During a sauna session, the pulse and stroke volume increase. Surface vessels dilate as blood is shunted from internal organs to the surface. Blood pressure usually remains the same or decreases during a session. Repeated sauna use helps decrease elevated blood pressure by enhancing elasticity of the arteries, removing toxins from the kidneys and helping to reduce excessive sympathetic nervous system activity.

Endocrine System. During sauna use, sympathetic inhibition causes decreased secretion of adrenal and thyroid hormones. This rests the glands. Blood sugar may decrease slightly. Insulin and glucagon secretion decrease. The removal of toxic substances benefits the entire endocrine system.

Kukkonen-Harjula and Kauppinen studied the effects of sauna bathing on thyroxin and TSH. They found that if one cools the body slowly after a session, there is no increase in these hormones. If cooling is fast, as in a cold shower, TSH increases. This is most likely simply a stress response and I do not recommend cold bathing after a sauna, in part for this reason.

Digestive System. Sympathetic inhibition may activate the digestive system during sauna use. Elimination of toxins from the liver and gall bladder may cause the need for a bowel movement after or even during a sauna session. Ulcers, colitis and intestinal infections may be helped greatly by repeated heating and sympathetic inhibition.

Skin. Saunas cleanse the skin from the inside and promote soft, pliable skin. Saunas also promote the healing of many skin conditions including acne, dermatitis and eczema. Others may include scarring, keloids, psoriasis and poisoning from too much sun exposure. Results may take several weeks to several months or even a year or more. However, some have reported excellent results with adult acne and other conditions after just a few days use of an infrared lamp sauna.

Sympathetic suppression and sweating cause the pores to open and decrease oil secretion by the sebaceous glands. Repeated heating is excellent to unblock clogged pores and reactivate skin that has become inactive and congested with toxins from synthetic clothing, skin care products and contact with toxic substances in bath water.

As for more technical aspects of the skin, a center in the preoptic region of the anterior hypothalamus controls temperature regulation. Heating causes vasodilation of all the skin vessels of the body and causes sweating. Vasodilation occurs by inhibition of sympathetic nerve fibers. The skin is also extremely sensitive to circulating epinephrine and norepinephrine. A decrease in these will also cause vasodilation.

According to Guyton's *Textbook of Medical Physiology*, sweating may cause additional vasodilation by a poorly-known mechanism that may involve bradykinin, a powerful vasodilator.

Effects of Saunas on the Oxidation Rate

Saunas have a normalizing effect on metabolism that will be reflected in measurements such as the oxidation rate as determined by a properly performed hair mineral analysis. The benefit occurs due to eliminating toxins and heavy metals that can cause either sluggish or excessive metabolic activity.

During a sauna session thyroid and adrenal activity tend to decrease slightly, causing a minor reduction in the metabolic rate. Slow oxidizers often suffer from sympathetic nervous system exhaustion and depleted adrenal and thyroid glands. They benefit from the rest afforded to the glands during sauna use and from the heating of the body, as their temperature is usually sub-normal. They need to use the sauna more often and for longer time periods than fast oxidizers, whose body temperature is already higher and who generally sweat more easily.

Saunas and Weight Loss

Weight loss or gain may occur from sauna sessions. Temporary weight loss occurs due to sweating. Reduction of edema due to improved circulation may also cause loss of water weight.

Some weight loss will also occur due to elimination of unhealthy tissue. At least one study by M. Imamura et al. found that patients with coronary risk factors lost significant weight after 15 minutes of sauna therapy daily for two weeks. Sauna therapy may also assist any weight loss program in the following ways:

• Repeated sauna use helps the body eliminate chemical toxins and heavy metals stored in fatty tissues. Inability to remove these substances as fatty tissues break down can be an important source of problems in weight loss programs.
• Fatty tissue often has poor circulation. Improving circulation with sauna therapy may help break down fat deposits.
• Repeated sauna use can help reduce cravings for sweets, starches or fatty foods. Often cravings are caused by toxic conditions and imbalances of the adrenals, thyroid, pancreas, liver and other organs.
• Improving the autonomic balance and body chemistry through the removal of toxic metals and chemicals can improve the digestion and absorption of nutrients. An important reason for obesity can be the desire to obtain more nutrients.
• Enhancing cellular metabolic processes can help burn fat calories more efficiently.

Weight gain may also occur in underweight individuals as glandular activity, digestion and absorption of nutrients improve.

Do Saunas Burn Calories?

Some claim that saunas burn hundreds of calories. I am not convinced of this. In a sauna session, the body does not have to burn calories to generate heat, as is the case with fever. Thus, I believe, many fewer calories are burned in a sauna than with a fever or with exercise. If one burned up to 600 calories in a 30-minute sauna session, as claimed, repeated sauna use would cause continuous weight loss. I have not observed this in practice.

Adding Energy To The Body

Saunas truly add energy to the body in the form of heat and, in the case of infrared saunas, light frequencies. "Evidence indicates that cells absorb photons and transform their energy into adenosine triphosphate or ATP." (*Interdisc. J. Rehab.,* Jan/Feb 2004)

Heating The Acupuncture Meridians

In oriental medicine, adding heat nourishes yang energy. This helps clear blockages and moves stagnant chi or energy. One acupuncturist described the effects of an infrared lamp sauna as similar to burning moxa on the skin to heat the meridians. Burning moxa is an acupuncture technique in which an herbal preparation is burned on the skin to increase yang or fiery energy.

Comparison of Sauna Effects With Those of Related Therapies

Fever Therapies, Hot Baths, Hot Tubs and Steam Baths Versus Sauna Hyperthermia

Inducing a fever has been used for hundreds of years as a method of healing many physical and even mental conditions. It is an excellent yet simple concept. The usual methods are to inject a person with pyrogenic or fever-producing bacteria, have one lie in a hot bath or wrap a person in hot towels or blankets. These methods share certain qualities with sauna hyperthermia, but are not the same in their effects, especially in the case of infrared sauna therapy.

In fever therapy due to the injection of bacteria, the body must produce the heat it requires to fight the infection. Producing this heat requires an increase in the metabolic rate with adrenal and thyroid activation via the sympathetic nervous system. This uses a lot of energy, so the therapy is exhausting and may therefore be less effective.

Also, activation of the sympathetic nervous system has a somewhat inhibitory effect on some aspects of the immune system.

In sauna hyperthermia, as well as hot baths or the use of hot towels, heat is supplied from without so the body does not have to expend energy to heat itself up. There is no appreciable increase in the metabolic or oxidation rate, no immune suppression and the therapy is less exhausting.

Hot baths, hot tubs and steam heat the body core very effectively by conduction. However, sweating is a little less intense due to the higher humidity. Also, temperature control is more difficult and delicate with hot baths and overheating can occur easily.

Detoxification can definitely occur with hot tubs and hot baths. One drawback to their repeated use is that chemical toxins are absorbed from the water itself and perhaps from the chemicals used to purify the water. Using steam, one absorbs chlorine and perhaps hundreds of other volatile organic chemicals present in tap water supplies. The humidity in hot tubs and steam rooms also supports the growth of many infection-causing bacteria.

Hot tubs and steam rooms heat the body from the outside only, as do hot air saunas. Infrared saunas heat from the inside, providing a more potent effect.

Electric Blankets Versus Saunas

Hyperthermia treatment for cancer may involve wrapping the patient in electric blankets, although at times a hot bath is used. Body temperature is increased to 105-106° F, very close to the temperature at which brain damage occurs. A problem with electric blankets is precisely controlling the temperature to make sure the patient does not overheat. Vital body functions must be carefully monitored. Extremely rapid release of toxins and cellular debris may overwhelm the eliminative organs. Dehydration is possible with blankets. Electric blankets also produce harmful electromagnetic fields.

Saunas do not raise the temperature nearly this high. However, they are safer, able to be done at home and usually do not require special and often costly monitoring. By gently and slowly reactivating the skin and the eliminative organs, sauna therapy also helps ensure that toxins will be eliminated safely.

Exercise Versus Saunas

Exercise vigorous enough to raise body temperature and produce copious sweating is exhausting for all but the most fit. Vigorous exercise requires extreme sympathetic nervous system activity. This inhibits immune system activity somewhat, can deplete the adrenal and thyroid glands and inhibits the organs of elimination such as the liver and kidneys. For these reasons, although one sweats with vigorous exercise, toxin elimination is less, we believe, than with sauna hyperthermia. Exercise is still helpful in moderation, but its effects are not at all the same as sauna therapy. More research is vitally needed regarding toxin elimination due to exercise versus that which occurs with infrared sauna use.

Fasting Versus Saunas

As health director for two and a half years at a fasting spa in Mexico, I worked with patients who came for weight loss and detoxification, among other reasons. The results were mainly disappointing.

I did not understand at the time that most people are far more depleted and toxic than when most of the classic texts were written about fasting. Especially long fasts often cause further nutritional depletion, although symptomatic improvement may occur. I do not recommend long fasts. Fasting for a day or two is fine. Juice fasting is less depleting than fasting on water alone.

Saunas can cause some mineral depletion. However, this can be avoided by replenishing minerals through diet or with kelp supplements. In our experience, sauna therapy is much safer than fasting and much more effective as well for deep tissue cleansing.

3
Heat Shock Proteins

"Forty months ago I was diagnosed with multiple myeloma with intense bone pain, anemia and spinal fractures. I was given three to nine months to live and began a metabolic cancer therapy program. It included three sauna sessions daily of 20-30 minutes each with an infrared lamp sauna.

Three years later, I have lost three inches of height from the cancer where my spine was fractured and I feel it when the weather changes. Otherwise, I am very well. The CEA (cancer marker) has dropped from 5.5 to 4.1.

I was found to have lead poisoning. The lead is gone, according to hair mineral testing and electrodermal testing. I am continuing the natural cancer therapy for a little longer and I know I will continue to use the infrared lamp sauna on a maintenance basis forever. - Mr. C.S., Anchorage, Alaska

An interesting area of medical research that may help explain some of the benefits of sauna therapy is that of *heat shock proteins* or HSPs. This chapter is a brief report on HSPs. Further research is needed to confirm or disprove the effects of sauna therapy on HSP production.

Heat shock proteins are special proteins found in all body cells that help regenerate damaged cells. They were first identified in the late 1970s and early 1980s in plant genetic research. Since then they have been found in all cells, from bacteria to humans.

Within minutes of undergoing certain kinds of stress, production of normal cell proteins ceases and instead HSPs are produced. It is as though the regular assembly line to produce proteins in the cells shuts down and another line starts up that regenerates the cell structures.

Once begun, HSP production can last up to nine days. Stressors that may induce HSP production include ischemia, influx of heavy metals or depletion of ATP (adensoine triphosphate). Others are protein degradation by drugs, inflammation, or mechanical or chemical stress such as oxidant stress.

One of the best inducers of the synthesis of heat shock proteins is heating the body several degrees.

"This stress response produces a transient rearrangement of cellular activities to cope with the stress period by protecting essential components within the cells so as to permit it to resume normal activity during recovery from the stress...Heat, both quantitatively and qualitatively, is one of the best inducers of heat stress proteins." *(Heat Shock Proteins in Myocardial Protection)*

Renaturation

Proteins are chains of amino acids that are bent, folded over and joined to each other in complex ways. *Denaturation* is the general term for damage to these complex structures. A simple example is cooking an egg. The egg protein is fairly liquid at room temperature. It becomes hardened in a few minutes when cooked. This is due to damage or denaturing of its protein structure.

HSPs help refold and reassemble damaged proteins. This is called *renaturation*. They also bind to heavily damaged proteins, preventing them from clumping or forming aggregates and shepherding them to areas of the cell where they can be degraded and recycled. By so doing, they can also block apoptosis or programmed cell death and can literally rescue cell proteins from stress-related damage. As a result of renaturing of proteins, all cell functions can be restored, including energy production, immune system activity, elimination, respiration and others.

A crude analogy is that HSPs function like the police who are called in the event of a disturbance. They clean up the mess and restore order. They arrive in minutes and stay around for a short while to make sure things are okay.

One may ask, why does the body not produce HSPs all the time? Possible reasons include: 1) they are not needed except in emergencies and 2) they use up large amounts of energy and nutrients that are better spent in other ways. It would be like having the police sit at one's door all the time when there is no need for them.

Heat Shock Therapy

Injecting HSPs can cause the body's T-cells to recognize a tumor and begin destroying it. However, HSPs are very specific for each person. Researchers investigating HSPs as a cancer therapy are having difficulty, therefore, producing HSPs that will work for everyone. Success in using heat shock proteins for cancer therapy so far occurs when the researchers grind up the patient's tumor, extract the patient's own HSPs and inject them back into the patient. Sauna therapy has the advantage of perhaps stimulating endogenous production of the exact HSPs each person requires without requiring knowledge of the patient's symptoms or condition.

I have not found research on the absolute temperature or temperature above basal temperature required to produce HSPs. However, to raise body temperature several degrees requires that one be in the second phase of a sauna session. This usually means spending at least 40 minutes of continuous time in an infrared lamp sauna. It would take longer in a far infrared sauna and longer still, perhaps an hour, in a hot air sauna.

Leaving the sauna every half hour or less, or drinking a lot of cold water during the sauna would likely impair production of HSPs. The less healthy the body, the easier it is to shock the system and therefore the more likely HSPs will be produced.

Raising the body temperature often causes fatigue. One should not leave a sauna just for this reason, as it may be an indicator of a shift in cellular metabolism associated with HSP production and cellular repair. To achieve excellent results, the heating needs to be repeated at least every few days to continue the process of cell repair.

A far infrared or infrared lamp sauna should produce more HSPs in a shorter time than a traditional sauna because heating occurs from inside the body. Perhaps this is one reason researchers report more effective detoxification with infrared saunas.

Analogous Concepts

Most readers know that if one places a frog in cool water and slowly adds hot water, the frog will stay put and burn to death. If, however, one drops a frog into hot water, the frog will immediately jump out of the water.

Our bodies degenerate slowly as they are chronically poisoned by heavy metals, toxic chemicals, bacteria and other toxins. However, an acute shock such as a fever or heating in a sauna may break the cycle by shifting the cells into a regenerative mode with the production of HSPs. This may be the value of fevers and acute illnesses. As people age or become debilitated, they are less able to produce a fever and their health status declines more rapidly as a result.

Other Metabolic Effects

Heat shock proteins help maintain the metabolic and structural integrity of cells. They can protect the heart, increase catalase activity and preserve high energy phosphates. They also increase antioxidant activity by enhancing glutathione production.

Research indicates that heat shock protein deficiency may be involved in prion diseases such as scrapie in sheep and bovine spongiform encephalitis (BSE) or mad cow disease in animals and humans. Prions are similar in some ways to heat shock proteins. Prions, in fact, protect organisms against ultra-violet radiation.

HSPs and Nutrition

HSP production appears to require the presence of extra nutrients, particularly zinc and manganese. Zinc is required for RNA transferase, an important enzyme involved in protein synthesis. Manganese is required for glycosyl transferase, a manganese-specific enzyme involved in glucose utilization.

Failure to produce HSPs in mad cow disease may be related to a manganese deficiency. Ken Purdy in Great Britain and other researchers found that cows with the disease had been doused with Phosmet, an organophosphate warble fly insecticide that damages prions, causing them to bind manganese. This may leave less manganese available for HSP production. The symptoms of mad cow disease are similar to the symptoms of 'manganese madness' found in manganese miners.

Deficiencies of zinc and manganese are widespread in the population due to food grown on mineral-depleted soils and refined food diets. Stress also rapidly depletes zinc. The best dietary sources of zinc are meats. Nuts and seeds are excellent dietary sources of manganese. A healthful diet and nutritional supplementation may enhance HSP production with sauna therapy.

Coley's Toxins and HSPs

Some readers may be familiar with the cancer toxins developed by William Coley, MD. Although not a mainstream cancer therapy, it was and is effective against some cases of cancer. Heat shock proteins are likely involved in this simple form of fever therapy.

Dr. Coley, a brilliant surgeon who worked at the Memorial Hospital in New York, later to be called Sloane-Kettering Memorial Hospital, reviewed a case of a man with a large round cell sarcoma on his neck. He had been declared hopeless when he developed a severe infection with erysipelas. Within a few days the huge malignant ulcer healed.

Coley's toxins are a combination of killed seratia marcescens and streptococcus pyogenes and their endotoxins. When injected, they can produce a very high fever. Within a few days, tumors can shrink and the cancer go into remission. Coley's toxins are still available at the Issels Treatment Center in Tijuana, Mexico.

Currently, researchers at UCLA are having some success injecting cancer patients with malaria, another disease that causes high fevers.

Sauna Protocol and HSPs

Usually, preheating an infrared light or far infrared sauna is unnecessary. However, for maximum HSP production preheating is helpful. It will raise body temperature faster to perhaps produce more HSPs. Further studies are needed to confirm the correct temperature and time required to produce HSPs.

4
Sauna Protocol

"I am 70 years old. After a terrible car accident two years ago, I was in constant pain. The infrared lamp sauna stops the pain. I will at times get up at 4 AM and do a sauna. After 30 minutes, the pain is gone. My sweat smells horrendous at times. This is probably due to the many medicines I took after the accident.

I was wearing a wig, but now my hair has come back as thick as when I was young. My nails, which were weak, have also become very strong, and I also have fewer wrinkles.

My husband noticed the joint pain in his ankles and hips went away. He walks better, he lost weight, he is happier and his golf game has improved. My husband and I plan to use the sauna regularly for the rest of our lives." - Mrs. A.W., Sun Lakes, Arizona

Types Of Saunas Used For Therapy

Any type of sauna can be used for therapy. However, the results will differ:

- *Traditional saunas* are those heated by a wood-burning or gas stove, hot rocks carried in from a fire, or an electric coil or gas heater.
- *Far infrared saunas* are heated by metallic or ceramic elements that emit a narrow spectum of mainly far infrared energy.
- *Infrared lamp saunas* use red, infrared heat lamps as their source of radiant heat. They provide a wide spectrum of infrared energy and some visible light as well.

Traditional Saunas

These are the familiar saunas found at health clubs, spas and in many homes. They are basically a room with a heater. Often the heater has a few heated rocks on top, onto which one can throw water to create steam in the sauna.

These saunas heat only the surface of the body mainly by *convection*. They operate at high temperatures of about 150-210° F. Healthy people can safely spend several hours daily in this type of sauna with supervision. These are the saunas used in L. Ron Hubbard's 'Purification

Rundown' and many similar detoxification programs. They were the only ones available at the time Mr. Hubbard developed his detoxification program.

L. Ron Hubbard pioneered the specific use of traditional saunas for drug and alcohol detoxification some 60 years ago. Later the program was expanded to include detoxification of toxic chemicals. The Foundation Of Science And Education has carefully researched and published the results of this program, which involves spending several hours per day in the sauna and taking niacin, an oil blend and other supplements under close medical supervision for several weeks or more. Over 500,000 people have been through the program with excellent results.

Many centers have sprung up in the United States and elsewhere offering the Hubbard Purification Rundown. The Hubbard method of sauna detoxification remains by far the most widely used protocol for sauna detoxification.

Far Infrared Saunas

Far infrared saunas were introduced about 30 years ago. They have from 6 to 12 or more ceramic or metallic heating elements in the walls of the sauna that emit mainly far infrared energy.

They heat the body mainly by *radiant energy*, warming the body from the inside as well as on the surface. Their energy penetrates into the body up to about 1.5 inches, according to their research. For this reason, they are effective at lower temperatures of about 130 °F. Research indicates they produce more effective tissue cleansing due to the penetration of the infrared rays. The cooler temperature is more comfortable for some people.

Far infrared saunas require less preheating and the units are more energy efficient than traditional saunas. *Up to three hours per day* spread out over several sessions may be safe for most healthy adults in this type of sauna. Power supplies and the ceramic or metallic elements can emit significant electromagnetic fields.

Infrared Lamp Saunas

Infrared lamp saunas are heated by three or more reddish-colored infrared heat lamps. These are often the common lamps sold at hardware stores. They emit a spectrum of frequencies including near, middle and a little far infrared energy. The energy peaks in the near infrared range. The lamps also emit some red, orange and yellow visible light.

The use of this type of sauna is a focus of this book. Only a few companies offer them at this time. These are listed in the resource section of this book and on our web site, *www.drlwilson.com*. This type of sauna can also be built fairly easily and plans are provided later in the book.

Infrared lamp saunas of the design we recommend penetrate deeper than the far infrared type, up to about three inches inside the body, we believe. They are also the most energy efficient and operate at the coolest temperature of about 110-115° F.

At this time, we recommend spending *a maximum of two hours per day* spread out over at least two sessions in an infrared lamp sauna. One may experience excessive detoxification symptoms or other effects of the light or infrared if one remains inside more than two hours.

Also, exercise caution regarding shining the lamps at the head. In most cases, the lamps should be pointed at the chest and abdomen. This is where the main organs of elimination and detoxification are located. Exposure to the head for 20 minutes or less appears safe, however, for most people. Exposure to the head for a limited time can also be very helpful for detoxification of the sinuses, ears, eyes, nasal passages and the brain.

The lamps do not emit significant electromagnetic fields. However, they produce intense heat and are somewhat delicate. One must sit or lie down 18" to 30" from the lamps. Also, one must place a wire mesh or other type of guard in front of the lamps to avoid accidentally touching them.

I am unaware of controlled studies comparing the effectiveness of the three different types of saunas. These studies are now in the planning stage. Some basic differences between the three types of saunas are summarized in the chart below.

Brief Comparison of The Three Types Of Saunas

	Traditional Sauna	*Far Infrared Sauna*	*Infrared Lamp Sauna*
Operating Temperature	150-210° F	120-140° F	110-115° F
Penetration of the Skin	Little	1.5 inches	3 inches
Preheating Time	30-60 min.	0-20 min	0-20 min
Infrared Benefits	Little	Some	Most
Color Therapy Benefits	None	None	Yes
Need To Rotate In The Sauna	No	No	Yes
Operating Expense	Higher	Medium	Lowest

Enclosures Versus Cabinets

In a sauna room or full-body enclosure, the head is inside the sauna. A sauna cabinet looks like a steam cabinet and the head is outside the sauna. A cabinet will be somewhat less effective than a full-body enclosure although one can still derive great benefit from it.

If possible, it is best to expose the head to the heat and infrared energy. Cabinets are better for those who have difficulty breathing in a sauna or who are claustrophobic. Many people who are claustrophobic can learn to tolerate and even become comfortable in a full-body enclosure.

If one has difficulty breathing with the head inside a sauna, one may open the door slightly or breathe through a piece of flexible 1" outside diameter plastic tubing that leads outside the enclosure through a ventilation opening. Enclosures are discussed in more detail in Chapter 12, Sauna Design.

Cost and Outfitting

Ready-made traditional and infrared saunas range from $2000-6000.00. Many are quite elaborate, with insulated, double-wall construction, built-in electronic controls and even built-in stereo systems. Custom built-in units are higher in price. At the time of this printing, we offer an inexpensive canvas-covered frame infrared lamp sauna for those with limited resources. Those with building experience can construct this sauna for several hundred dollars or less. Basic plans are provided in Appendix D. See our website, *www.drlwilson.com* for details regarding companies that sell infrared lamp saunas.

One can use a traditional sauna at a health club, clinic or health center. However, this is inconvenient because it should be used daily or even twice daily. Having to drive back and forth is not optimal.

To outfit a sauna for therapy, one may wish to add on top or inside a boom box or small sound system for sound therapy. An inside clock or timer is also helpful. Infrared lamps may be added to traditional or far infrared saunas to provide extra infrared radiant energy and color therapy.

Steam

Some people like steam in their sauna. Advantages of steam are that it raises the temperature in a hot air sauna and thus helps induce sweating and other effects. Steam also feels good to some people. Throwing water on hot rocks adds negative ions that may make breathing easier.

The disadvantages of steam are that the added humidity causes one to sweat a little less than when steam is not present. Also, the added heat is difficult to tolerate for many people. Most important, one will absorb some chemicals that are in the water that is used to make the steam. These include chlorine, fluorides and possibly hundreds of volatile organic chemicals.

Steam is not added to infrared saunas as it not part of the design. Never throw water on the hot lamps of an infrared lamp sauna.

When to Use a Sauna

For greatest safety and healing effects, *wait one or better two hours after meals before a sauna session. Also, first thing in the morning and the last thing at night are best for sauna use.* At these times, one is most relaxed. This produces the greatest detoxification effect. Activities, exercise and distractions in the middle of the day often stimulate the sympathetic nervous system and interfere with the sauna's healing effects. In a healing facility, any time of the day is fine as long as it is one or two hours after a meal.

How Often to Use a Sauna

Saunas are generally very safe for most people. However, very imbalanced tissue levels of calcium, magnesium, sodium or potassium could make sauna use more hazardous. One could sweat out enough of a vital mineral such as potassium to cause heart arrhythmias or other metabolic problems. I have not seen this in practice. However, it is possible.

The decision of how often to use saunas depends on the setting. In the residential detoxification programs that follow the L. Ron Hubbard approach, one may spend up to five hours daily in a traditional sauna. I recommend Mr. Hubbard's book, *Clear Body, Clear Mind* for more details on this type of sauna therapy.

The present book focuses on home use of infrared saunas without direct medical supervision. For these programs, most people can use a sauna once or twice daily. Weekly sauna use is more for maintenance, not therapy. Specific cautions and contraindications are discussed at the end of this chapter.

If you suspect serious tissue mineral imbalances, limit the duration of sauna sessions at first to a maximum of 20 minutes until the imbalances improve. Also, begin with fewer sessions per week and shorter sessions if very debilitated. For the very frail, one can begin with a milder infrared experience by keeping the door open or sitting in front of infrared lamps without an enclosure.

I have used hair mineral analysis from a laboratory that does not wash the hair to assess electrolyte imbalances that may affect the duration and frequency of sauna sessions. Hair analysis is a tissue test and a much better way to assess actual stores of minerals in most cases than blood or urine tests. Those with low hair calcium and magnesium and elevated hair sodium and potassium generally require and prefer one sauna session daily. However, those with elevated hair calcium and magnesium levels and low hair sodium and potassium levels usually do better with twice or even more sessions daily. For more details on the use of hair mineral testing to assess potentially hazardous electrolyte imbalances, see Appendix A.

How Long to Remain in a Sauna

This depends on your health status and whether you have an acute infection. When an acute infection is present, such as a cold, flu or pneumonia, more frequent and shorter sauna sessions are often best. This is also a good idea during a healing or purification reaction. Refer to the section later in this chapter titled 'Sauna Protocol For Acute Infections'.

The remainder of this section concerns sauna protocol when one does not have an acute infection. The duration of a sauna session may be based on time, heart rate elevation or temperature elevation.

Time. Most people can begin with 20 minutes in a sauna. Limit the first week's sessions to a maximum of 30 minutes per session. This is to avoid too many healing reactions. The duration of a session can increase up to 60 minutes total time after several weeks to several months, depending on your condition. *The total time spent per day in a hot air sauna should not exceed five hours. In a far infrared sauna, do not exceed three hours and do not exceed two hours daily in an infrared lamp sauna.* This is important because it is possible to overdo sauna therapy.

When beginning sauna therapy, many people do not sweat properly. As a result, one can overheat if the body cannot adequately handle the heat. If this occurs, one may turn red, the pulse may race and body temperature can rise quickly, making one feel uncomfortable. If overheating occurs, begin with shorter sessions. With repeated sauna sessions, the skin becomes more active. Temperature regulation and vital mineral retention improve. Then one can safely increase the duration of sauna sessions.

Heart Rate. An increase in the pulse is due to heating the body, not a sympathetic response as in exercise. As core body temperature rises, the pulse will increase. An increase of *up to 50% above the resting pulse* is safe unless a heart condition necessitates keeping it lower.

Body Temperature. The basal temperature will usually rise a few degrees if you stay in a sauna for 30 minutes or more. An increase of *up to 4° F* is safe for most people and excellent for healing. This much of an increase, however, is not always necessary to achieve desired results. To experiment with this, take your oral temperature on entering the sauna and check it every five minutes or so. Oral temperature will read one degree lower than rectal temperature.

As the body acclimates to saunas, sweating can increase fourfold and temperature regulation becomes more efficient. The core temperature may not rise quite as much, although one will still receive benefits from the sauna. Temperature should not be allowed to rise beyond about 103° F.

Sauna Danger Signals

If the heart starts racing, if sweating stops or if there is difficulty breathing, end the session. If you develop persistent pain, end the session.

How Much Sauna Therapy

Sauna *therapy*, as compared with recreational use, is for a limited time. In our experience, most people should stay on a daily sauna therapy program for at least two years to remove the bulk of their toxic metals, toxic chemicals and chronic infections. For a degenerative illness such as cancer, at least two years of therapy are needed.

For more acute conditions, such as a chemical exposure, a year or less may suffice. However, most people are carrying a large load of toxic chemicals and metals of which they are completely unaware. When the intent is to heal a chronic condition such as an injury, continue therapy for at least two months after symptoms disappear.

Replenishing Minerals

One will sweat out some minerals during a sauna session that need to be replaced. *Add a teaspoon or more of sea salt and up to one or two tablespoons of kelp granules to your diet. Those who do not like the taste of kelp may use 12-15 kelp tablets or 3-6 larger kelp capsules.*

Most people can add two or three teaspoons of kelp daily to the diet for a year or even two. This is very adequate to replace the beneficial minerals lost during sweating.

Kelp is an excellent and inexpensive source of many minerals. Other mineral supplements do not contain as many minerals. Most people handle kelp well. A few who are hyperthyroid cannot take kelp and will need to use other mineral supplement. 'Natural' mineral supplements, including kelp, contain some toxic metals. Kelp, however, contains a lot of *alginates*, substances that bind toxic metals and prevent their absorption into the body. I do not recommend any other seaweeds such as dulse, nori or others as they do not contain as much alginates.

Many doctors recommend various mineral cocktails before or after sauna use. I do not recommend these at all. Avoid drinking most juices, Gatorade, Recharge or other mineral replacement drinks. A few of these drinks are okay. However, most are very sugary, yin (cold and too expansive in Chinese medicine) and will diminish the benefits of sauna therapy. Eat a diet of natural foods, preferably organically grown. Drink good quality spring water if you would like to obtain additional minerals. Recall from Chapter 2 that mineral retention will improve as the body acclimates to sweating.

Mineral Replacement and Biological Transmutation. Dr. Louis Kervan is the author of *Biological Transmutations*. This is a fascinating subject that calls into question some deeply held beliefs about physical chemistry and the nature of chemical elements. Dr. Kervan studied workers in the Sahara Desert who sweated out far more potassium than they replaced, with no adverse effects. He theorized that a transmutation occurs, converting sodium to potassium in an endothermal reaction, which also helped them handle the heat. The same phenomenon may occur in saunas, as extremely few negative health effects have been reported for sweat lodges and saunas used by millions of people for hundreds of years.

After presenting the mathematical heat calculations, Dr. Kervan wrote:

"I came to the conclusion that it was sodium which, disappearing to become potassium, created an endothermal reaction, thus causing heat to be absorbed. Hence, by instinct, one consumes more salt in dry and hot country. This is why salt is so important in Africa, the Middle East, etc., where caravans travel up to 1000 kilometers to bring back salt."

"The transmutation from sodium to potassium was confirmed by another experiment made in a more arid part of the Sahara... in a physiology laboratory. A man making a major physical effort during three hours, in a temperature of 39° C with a humidity of 60%, would experience an increase of three times his usual rate of potassium in proportion to sodium in his urine." (*Biological Transmutations*, p. 28)

Before a Sauna Session

Wait at least one, and preferably two hours after eating, before entering a sauna. Also, drink 8-16 ounces of preferably spring water. Children may drink less. Light clothing may be worn in a wood, gas-fired or electric coil-heated sauna. No clothing is usually worn in an infrared sauna, although a skimpy bathing suit is fine.

If using a hot air sauna, set the thermostat to about 160° F and enter when it has reached that temperature. In a far infrared sauna, set the thermostat to about 125°F and enter as soon as one turns it on. This allows maximum exposure to the beneficial infrared rays. When the temperature inside reaches 120-125° F, open the ventilation louvers or open the door about 1/4" so the sauna does not get hotter. This will keep the far infrared elements operating the entire sauna session to maximize the beneficial rays.

In an infrared lamp sauna, follow a similar procedure. Enter as soon as one turns on the lamps. As the temperature reaches 110-115° F, open the door about 1/4" so the temperature remains at this level. One must rotate every few minutes in an infrared lamp sauna to heat the body evenly, assuming the lamps are on only one side of the sauna. One may also preheat a far infrared or infrared lamp sauna for 10-20 minutes to achieve slightly higher temperatures. This is advisable for patients with a chronic illness such as cancer, as it may help produce more heat shock proteins.

Preparing A Sauna For Therapy

	Traditional Sauna	Far Infrared Sauna	Infrared Lamp sauna
Set Thermostat At:	About 160° F.	About 125° F.	About 115° F.
Preheat?	Yes, up to at least 130° F.	If desired, or enter as soon as you turn it on	If desired, or enter as soon as you turn it on

During And After A Sauna Session

Wipe off sweat with a small towel and sit on a second small towel. Spread a large towel on the floor. Spend the time in the sauna visualizing or relaxing. Odors or sensations may occur during a session. If an odor is objectionable, open the door for a few seconds to let in fresh air. Most will pass quickly. Most bodily sensations are completely benign. Relax, breathe deeply and attempt to continue the session unless extremely uncomfortable or faint. Most sensations will pass quickly as toxic substances are released and the body rebalances itself. At times, a healing reaction can last for several days or even weeks. However, it is often best to continue sauna therapy during the reaction to help it resolve faster. Healing reactions are discussed in detail in Chapter 11.

I recommend exposing the palms of the hands directly to the heat and infrared if one is in an infrared sauna. This will enhance the effects of the session. Many acupuncture and reflex points are close to the surface on the hands.

When a sauna session is finished, shower with cool or warm, but preferably not hot water. If possible, do not wait long after a sauna before showering, as some toxins will be reabsorbed. If you cannot shower, then towel off the sweat after the session.

Rinse off the two small sweat-filled towels in the shower until they do not smell and hang them up to dry. Brush the skin all over with a loofa or skin brush, including the scalp and face. One will be very clean. If possible, avoid using soap or shampoo, or putting anything on the skin. Drink 8-16 ounces of spring water and *rest lying down or sitting down for at least 10 minutes* before resuming daily activities. *Resting is very important!* You may eat after resting. If you are also using coffee enemas for detoxification, use the sauna before doing a coffee enema.

While resting after the sauna, one may do a short practice borrowed from Total Body Modification. To recenter, place the fingers of the right hand on the right groin area and the left hand on the left frontal sinus on the forehead. Hold for five seconds or until your breathing relaxes. Then place the fingers of the left hand on the left groin area and the right hand on the right side of the frontal sinus. Hold for five seconds or until your breathing relaxes.

You will also need to rest more during the day while on a sauna therapy program. The changes caused by the program continue throughout the day. You may suddenly experience fatigue, headaches, faintness or other symptoms as toxins are released. Usually, lying down for 15 to 30 minutes will help immensely, allowing the body to process the changes with less interference. If at all possible, arrange your schedule so there is time for rest periods during the day. Resting facilitates detoxification by reducing sympathetic nervous system activity.

Cleaning the Sauna. The floor of a wood sauna should be cleaned once a week to once a month to prevent or reduce rotting. Oxiclean™, a readily available non-toxic cleaner, is excellent to remove bacteria and mold. The walls and ceiling usually need cleaning less often.

Those who operate detoxification centers will attest to the foul odors and at times stains that occur due to sweating. Max Gerson, MD reported that after each patient left his cancer clinic the walls required repainting due to persistent toxic odors.

Supervision

Supervision is essential during sauna therapy, moreso if one is ill. This is not a do-it-yourself therapy. As metals and organic chemicals are released, healing reactions will occur. Even experienced physicians can become discouraged, disoriented or frightened. It is most helpful to have someone to check with, at least by telephone, at these times.

This book provides basic information about sauna therapy. However, healing reactions and circumstances may be different for each individual. I have included my own experiences in Chapter 14 as examples of the kinds of reactions that may occur during sauna therapy. If at all possible, when doing sauna therapy work with a practitioner or someone familiar with healing reactions.

Relaxation

Detoxification requires a relaxed nervous system. Relax before entering the sauna. If tense, a drop or two of rose, lavender or another relaxing essential oil in the sauna may be helpful. Place it on a small plate or surface. A diffuser should not be needed.

One may also begin a sauna session listening to relaxing music. Avoid working, studying or talking while in the sauna. A massage before or after a sauna session is excellent. A foot massager or foot roller can also be used in a sauna.

Maintaining a relaxed lifestyle throughout a sauna therapy program will greatly assist detoxification and healing. Avoid strenuous activity, including heavy exercise, strenuous travel or very long work hours. Ask for cooperation from family members and friends during the program.

Sauna Therapy During Acute Infections

Acute infections include colds, the flu, earaches, or active infection anywhere in the body. Symptoms may include fever, aches and pains, inflammation or diarrhea. During an acute infection, prolonged sauna therapy is less helpful. The body is focused on resolving the infection. Extensive detoxification or other intense sauna effects can interfere with healing the acute condition.

It is best to have shorter sauna sessions when an acute infection is present. Ten to fifteen-minute sessions are sufficient, repeated six to nine times per day. Be sure to rest in between these short sessions. Also, if you are using an infrared lamp sauna, focus more energy on the infected area. For a stomach flu, for instance, spend more time with the lamps focused on the front of the body. For a sinus infection, move the front of the head closer to the lamps. Heat is beneficial, so preheat the sauna to about 100°. Once the infection passes, return to the regular sauna therapy protocol.

A person's regular nutritional supplements may also be unnecessary and perhaps harmful during acute infections. Chapter 9 contains a more complete discussion of supplement recommendations for infections.

Cautions and Contraindications

One should have an attendant or friend nearby when doing sauna therapy if one is very heat-sensitive, has multiple sclerosis, diabetes, a heart condition or has used psychotropic drugs in the past. The following conditions may require extra care when using a sauna:

Breast Implants. No problems have been reported. Wear a bra or bikini top if you are concerned about them, as this clothing will stop the penetration of the infrared into this area.

Children. Children under about six years old should avoid sauna use. Their sweat glands are less developed than adults. Their bodies also have a higher water content than adults and thus they can dehydrate more easily. Far infrared may also be harmful for children under five.

High Blood Pressure. Sauna use generally does not raise blood pressure. However, begin with shorter sessions and check blood pressure every ten minutes if you are concerned.

Dental Amalgams. You may use a sauna even if you have silver amalgam dental fillings or other dental metals in your mouth. We recommend having amalgams replaced when possible with safer dental materials. The exception is while one has an active cancer condition, at which time amalgam removal can be quite dangerous.

Past Use of LSD or other Psychedelic Drugs. Flashbacks can occur, including full-blown LSD trips, as stored drugs are mobilized from tissue storage sites. If at all possible, have an attendant or friend present during sauna use.

Multiple Sclerosis. Patients may be extremely heat sensitive. Begin with shorter sessions and have an attendant present in case extreme weakness should occur. However, some doctors report saunas can be very useful for multiple sclerosis.

Respiratory Conditions. Some experience breathing difficulty in saunas. Often this will improve as one acclimates to sweating. Be sure to sit up comfortably and breathe slowly and deeply. If uncomfortable, open the door about 1/2" to let in cooler air. One may also breathe through a 1" diameter plastic tube leading outside the sauna through a ventilation opening.

Lymph Node Removal. If one has had lymph nodes removed, for example during breast cancer surgery, circulation in the arms will be slightly impaired. In our experience, sauna therapy is still excellent. Begin with only 15 minutes in the sauna to see if there is any problem with circulation.

Diabetes. Begin with less time in the sauna and observe any unusual changes in blood sugar. Saunas do not significantly increase the metabolic rate. Nor do they tend to increase the blood sugar level or utilization of glucose. A decrease in blood sugar in the sauna is possible as sympathetic nervous system activity is inhibited.

Prostheses, Silicone Implants or Metallic Pins or Rods in the Body. These could heat up excessively in an infrared sauna, although I have not observed this. Begin with less time in the sauna, becoming aware of any unusual sensations in the area of the prostheses or pins.

Jewelry. Wearing jewelry is not advisable. It might become hot enough to cause a burn.

Medication. Rarely, heating the body may alter the properties or effects of a medication. This could occur with corticosteroids, for example. Consult the prescribing physician if this is a concern.

Menstruation. Menstruating women may experience a temporary increase in menstrual flow due to heating the low back. One need not avoid sauna use, but be aware that it may occur.

Pregnancy. To be on the safe side, if pregnant spend no more than 10 minutes at a time in a sauna and have a maximum of four sessions per week.
Exposure to intense heat during the first trimester of pregnancy may slightly increase the risk of birth defects. However, in a 1988 paper, Dr. K. Vaha-Eskeli and R. Ekkola of the Department of Obstetrics and Gynecology at the University of Turku reported that:

> "Up to 90% of pregnant women in Finland regularly visit the sauna until the expected time of delivery... Finnish women are confident that the sauna and pregnancy are compatible, a view that contrasts with many opinions abroad." (This statement refers to traditional hot air saunas. I am unaware of studies of pregnancy and infrared saunas.)

Saunas and Breastfeeding. While it is probably safe, I am unaware of studies of whether toxins released during a sauna therapy program could find their way into breast milk. Until good studies are performed, it would be prudent to reduce or avoid intense sauna therapy while one is breastfeeding a baby. The only exception would be if it is a matter of dire importance to the mother, such as in a case of cancer or another serious condition. In this instance, the risk of releasing some toxins into the breast milk may be worthwhile if the baby does not show any signs or symptoms of colic or other distress due to breastfeeding in this situation.

For Men. The testicles should remain cooler than the rest of the body. Technically, it may be best to avoid direct infrared irradiation of the testicles if you are concerned about fertility, as the testicles are somewhat heat sensitive. A 1988 paper from Finland reported no evidence that hot air sauna use decreases sperm count in men. However, infrared may have a more powerful effect due to deep tissue heating.

Young Children. Spend no more than 20 minutes in a sauna, always accompanied by an adult. Under age six, avoid sauna use.

The Elderly. Age per se is not a contraindication for sauna use. One's health status is far more important. In Finland, nearly 90% of those over age 80 are reported to be using saunas regularly. Dr. Jonathan Halperin, professor of internal medicine at Mount Sinai Medical Center in New York wrote: "Moderate sauna use is safe for most older people, but diabetics and anyone being treated for heart or circulatory conditions should check with their doctor, particularly if they are taking medications." (reported by Dorothy Bernstein, *Good Housekeeping Magazine*)

Maximum Duration of Sessions. A basically healthy person should spend no more than five hours per day in a hot air sauna, replacing water and electrolytes and taking a break at least every hour. One can use a far infrared sauna up to three hours a day, provided one replaces water and electrolytes and takes a break every hour. One can safely use an infrared lamp sauna up to two hours per day provided one replaces water and electrolytes and takes at least two breaks. Two to three shorter sessions are preferable, spread out through the day.

If one is debilitated, begin a program with less time in the sauna.

Dangers of Mineral Imbalances. Some authorities recommend specific electrolyte replacement drinks. In our experience, consuming extra sea salt and kelp are usually sufficient to replace electrolytes. Drinking quality spring water also helps replace vital trace minerals. Use extra caution if one has very low hair tissue levels of calcium, magnesium, sodium or potassium until these levels improve.

Elimination of Medications. During sauna therapy one will eliminate residues of prescription and over-the-counter medications, often taken years ago. These medications can include stimulants, sedatives, antibiotics, novocaine, chemotherapy and many others. Their release from storage can cause temporary effects similar to the action of the drug when first taken.

For example, eliminating stored antibiotics might damage the intestinal flora temporarily, causing some diarrhea or constipation. Eliminating stored Novocaine can cause temporary numbness of the face or jaw. Usually these effects pass quickly as the residues are excreted.

Moving Slowly. Sauna accidents can occur by slipping on wet floors, moving too quickly or with jerky movements, and drinking alcohol that impairs your judgment. Always move slowly and cautiously in a sauna. Avoid slippery surfaces by placing a towel on the floor.

Also move slowly and cautiously in and around the shower after a sauna session. The effects of heating will still be present and one may be light-headed and slightly faint from the sauna session.

Wheelchairs and Crutches. Saunas may be used by those on crutches or in wheelchairs. Metallic parts of wheelchairs and crutches, especially if dark-colored, may heat up excessively inside a sauna. Exercise care not to touch them or wrap them with electrical tape. Enclosure modifications for handicap use of a sauna are discussed in Chapter 12, Sauna Design.

Meals. Avoid eating for an hour or two before sauna therapy and avoid heavy meals two hours before using a sauna. A lot of blood is required to digest a meal, particularly a large one. The effect of a sauna is to shunt blood away from the internal organs to the skin. This will interfere with digestion and could cause cramping.

Also avoid sauna therapy when very hungry, although a sauna first thing in the morning is fine. At other times of the day, it is fine to use a sauna two to five hours after eating a meal. It is fine to eat 15 minutes after sauna therapy.

Alcohol. Saunas and alcohol do not mix! Alcohol can cause a false sensation of how hot you are, allowing you to remain in the sauna too long. Also, you may fall asleep, which is not a good idea. Carlton Hollander, in his book *How to Build a Sauna*, wrote:

"Alcohol is definitely not recommended prior to a sauna, since it works as a depressant, with a quick flash of energy leading into a state where the blood is moving slowly and the nerve endings are literally shutting down. The alcohol tends to detract from the total benefit of the sauna experience."

Talking, Reading or Working During Sauna Use. Some people wish to use the time in a sauna for working, phoning or reading. This can reduce the detoxification effects of the sauna by shifting the body somewhat into a more active or sympathetic state. While okay, it is preferable to use the time during a sauna session for meditating, visualizing or just relaxing.

Sensory Nerve Damage. Exercise caution in a sauna if you have had an injury, illness or skin graft that caused sensory nerve damage so you do not feel heat. Otherwise, you could stay in a sauna too long, which could cause burns or other difficulties.

Overdoing Sauna Therapy. Many people believe that if 20-30 minutes in a sauna is excellent, more must be better. Others enjoy the sessions so much they extend them excessively. Still others build saunas with more than one overhead heat lamp, which is not recommended.

Overdoing is not likely to do permanent damage. It will, however, cause healing reactions that can be intense. A few have become discouraged this way. It is important to begin with sauna sessions no longer than 20 minutes. Within a few weeks to a few months, the length of sessions may be increased. Sauna therapy is powerful and must be approached with common sense and caution, especially when beginning.

Pets. Do not bring pets into a sauna, either for therapy or companionship. Short exposure is probably fine for most animals. However, dogs and cats do not sweat as easily and may overheat in a sauna.

One may use a single red infrared heat lamp to treat an infection, abscess or other local condition in an animal. Follow the instructions in Appendix F regarding single lamp therapy. This should be safe as one is not raising the animal's core body temperature.

When I mentioned to a veterinarian that I was interested in infrared lamp therapy, he quickly told me he uses a red heat lamp on every animal he operates on to enhance healing after surgery.

Danger Signals in a Sauna. While very rare, one could experience heat stroke if one remains too long in a sauna. Danger signals are a rapid elevation of body temperature, cessation of sweating, a racing heart, extreme redness of the skin and feeling extremely faint. If any of these occur, end the session right away.

Claustrophobia. A large window or even a wall made of glass helps many people who are claustrophobic. Keeping the door slightly open reduces the heat, but may be easier to tolerate. Finally, in our experience, many claustrophobic people can learn to tolerate and even enjoy saunas with a little practice.

Burning From Heat Lamps. This is unlikely, as one will feel a burning sensation before an actual burn occurs. Some reddening of the skin normally occur with any infrared sauna and will go away within an hour. If the lamps burn, sit further away from the lamps and rotate more often. If your skin is very sensitive, unscrew one lamp or place a piece of metal window screen in the lamp guard to reduce the intensity of the lamp.

Using a sauna with breast implants. I have not had any reports of problems using a near infrared lamp sauna if one has breast implants. If you are concerned, wear a bikini top or bra in the sauna, and this will protect the area from the penetrating infrared light. In fact, anyone can wear a bikini bathing suit in a near infrared lamp sauna. This reduces the benefits of the sauna very little.

Eye sensitivity to the reddish heat lamps. Very rarely, someone says the red light bothers their eyes. Wear sunglasses if this occurs.

Skin cancer. Near infrared lamp sauna therapy does not cause skin cancer. In fact, it may help reduce it. However, the light may be irritating to a skin cancer. If this occurs, cover the skin cancer with a bandage or a piece of clothing. This will stop most of the infrared rays.

5
Detoxification

" I was diagnosed with Chronic Fatigue Syndrome, Epstein-Barr Virus Syndrome, acid reflux and high levels of candida albicans. I began to feel better after just five sessions of sauna therapy and continue to feel better after three months of its use.

I believe the sauna may be reducing my viral load. I also have less acid reflux and generally feel stronger. My husband built a "closet sauna" in the small building behind our house according to the specifications in your book. The temperature only gets to 95-100 degrees. Regardless, I am able to sweat quite a bit. I am so thankful for this information." - Mrs. R. H., Tallahassee, Florida

Saunas offer many benefits. Facilitating detoxification is probably the most unique and essential. This chapter discusses some mechanisms of sauna detoxification as well as many other topics related to detoxification.

The Philosophy of Detoxification

The idea that toxic substances cause disease is very ancient. It is mentioned in Greek and Roman medical texts, and in older writings as well. Ancient Chinese medical writings speak of 'harmful chi' and contain other references to toxins that cause illness. Herbal medicine and natural healing methods have emphasized toxin removal for thousands of years. Baths, enemas, poultices, emetics, laxatives, purgatives, skin brushing, cleansing diets and other methods for eliminating poisons are integral parts of these sciences.

Conventional medicine has not paid attention to most of this knowledge, perhaps in part because many allopathic drugs are themselves toxic substances. In fact, however, conventional medicine emphasizes the role of biological toxins in human disease. This includes the microorganisms themselves, and their endo-and exotoxins. We must be extremely grateful for the enormous contribution of modern allopathic medicine in understanding the role of biological toxins in human health and disease.

It is important to note that prescription and over-the-counter drugs may remain in the body for 30 years or more. Most physicians and pharmacists are unaware of the persistent nature of pharmaceuticals in the body. Upon undertaking a detoxification program, medication taken years before may be eliminated. One may smell or taste it, or experience pharmacologic effects as the drug is liberated from tissues and circulates in the blood until removed.

Toxins may be naturally-occurring or man-made substances. They may be introduced from outside the body and include metals, organic chemicals, ionizing radiation and microorganisms of many varieties. They may also be generated within. This is sometimes called *autointoxication*. Impaired digestion, fermentation of sugars and carbohydrates, putrefaction of protein and the end products of metabolism the body cannot eliminate are important endogenous sources of toxic chemicals. Also, bacteria and fungi may produce powerful endo- and exotoxins anywhere in the body.

To summarize this brief introduction to detoxification, toxin elimination is a valid and useful science. As we shall see, sauna therapy can serve as a very safe, powerful and cost-effective healing modality for toxin elimination.

Sauna Detoxification Mechanisms

Heating the Body

Heating the body several degrees causes greatly increased circulation as the body attempts to maintain its basal temperature. This helps to dislodge toxins, especially from hard-to-reach areas such as teeth, bones and sinuses.

Since many pathological microorganisms are heat-sensitive, the sauna's heat may weaken them or could kill some of them. Cells damaged by toxic metals and chemicals are weaker than normal cells. Heating also hastens their death, assisting the body to remove any metals or chemicals trapped inside.

Hyperthermia is one of the few methods available for eliminating radiation from the body. Mutated or otherwise radiation-damaged cells are often more sensitive to heat. Repeated sauna use, especially with infrared saunas, may selectively help to destroy them so they do not reproduce. This prevents the multiplication of mutated cells. Destroying the cells also allows the body to more rapidly remove radioactive isotopes lodged within these cells. Far infrared and infrared lamp saunas may be more effective for this task as their heat penetrates more deeply.

Many people today have a low body temperature. Heating the body a few degrees may greatly assist to normalize enzymatic activity, enhancing all cellular functions including detoxification. Applying external heat in a sauna is also one of the best ways to inhibit the sympathetic nervous system, which in turn is excellent to enhance the activity of the eliminative organs.

Skin Activation

The skin is a major eliminative organ. However, wearing clothing and exposure to toxic chemicals in synthetic clothing, skin care products and bath water congest and deactivate the skin in almost everyone. Sauna therapy brings large amounts of blood to the skin that rejuvenates and reactivates the skin as a major eliminative channel.

Sweating

Sweating is a superb method of eliminating many types of toxins. It spares the liver and kidneys and, for this reason, is safer than many other methods. Most people, especially slow metabolizers and those who are older or have sedentary lifestyles, do not sweat easily. Lead, cadmium, mercury, radioactive particles, pesticides and many other organic chemicals can be eliminated through the skin.

Most substances eliminated through the kidneys can be eliminated by the skin. Sweating thus helps relieve the burden of toxin elimination that falls to the kidneys. This rests the kidneys and assists their regeneration and ability to detoxify.

Dr. Michael Lyon, MD, of the Cline Medical Center Hyperthermic Detoxification Program wrote:

"Since sweat is manufactured from lymph, toxins present in the lymph fluid will exit the body through the sweat. Because the liver and kidneys are not required for this process, these organs are largely unburdened by hyperthermic therapy and toxins are able to leave the body even when liver or kidney function is impaired."

Note that sweating in a sauna is likely much more helpful for detoxification than sweating during exercise for two reasons:

- Saunas conserve the body's energy by providing the heat externally. This frees energy for detoxification.
- Sweating with exercise powerfully activates the sympathetic nervous system. This reduces the activity of the eliminative organs - the liver, kidneys and colon.

Exercise is still beneficial, however, especially for oxygenation of the tissues.

Hot and Dry (Yang) Effects

Sauna therapy, especially infrared sauna therapy, is a yang therapy. Yin and yang denote qualities of the body that are cold or hot, expanded or contracted. This is a central concept in Chinese medicine and can become quite complex. The following is a simplification.

Most bodies today are yin according to Chinese medical diagnosis. Perhaps this is because almost all chemical toxins and heavy metals are yin. Radiation toxicity, dramatically increased in the past 50 years, is extremely yin and affects everyone negatively. All therapy methods are yin, yang or some combination.

Yin Detoxification. *Yin detoxification methods flush toxins with cool and watery energy.* They slow down an overheated metabolism. They include raw foods, fruit and juice fasts and vegetarian diets. Other yin therapies are vitamin C therapy, radiation therapy, cold baths, some enemas and colonic irrigation, anti-inflammatory drugs, antibiotics and most other pharmaceuticals, many herbs and some acupuncture techniques. Most vitamins are yin, especially water-soluble ones. Fat-soluble vitamins and glandulars are more yang.

Yang Detoxification. *Yang methods heat, activate and contract the body to enhance toxin removal.* These include saunas, coffee enemas, therapy with red and infrared light, and hot baths. They also include diets with kelp, sea salt, meats and cooked vegetables, especially root vegetables. For a more yang diet, avoid yin foods such as sugar and fruit juices in particular. Reduce the amount fruit and uncooked foods in general.

As more people have become yin, they require more yang therapies. This may be a reason more problems are arising with antibiotic overuse and vegetarian diets. Understanding yin and yang detoxification helps explain why a particular therapy works for one but not for another. The principle applies to conventional as well as holistic therapies. It also helps explain why a therapy that worked 50 years ago may not work as well today.

In my experience, yang therapies are appropriate for more than 90% of adults. The others, whose bodies are more yang, require modifying the recommendations in this book with more raw food, less animal products, fewer saunas and more vegetable juices.

Assessing Yin and Yang Conditions. On a mineral analysis, elevated tissue calcium and magnesium with low tissue sodium and potassium is roughly indicative of a yin state. The opposite pattern is associated with a more yang condition. In general, mineral analysis correlates closely with traditional Chinese pulse and tongue diagnosis.

Some practitioners use face diagnosis to assess yin and yang conditions. I believe this is less reliable because several patients were diagnosed yang with face diagnosis while mineral analysis revealed an extreme yin condition. Many who appear yang are not. They are merely toxic and under temporary stress. When the toxins are released and stress diminishes, they become yin.

Improving Circulation

Many people, especially those who are older, more sedentary or slow metabolizers, have poor circulation that impairs detoxification. Sauna use is one of the finest way to improve circulation without requiring a great expenditure of energy. Enhancing circulation forces more blood through the eliminative organs and can help eliminate toxic minerals and chemicals that deposit in areas of poor circulation.

Strengthening The Parasympathetic Nervous System

Sympathetic nervous system activity, related to the fight-or-flight response, is catabolic. It breaks down tissue and increases thyroid and adrenal activity to respond to stress. Stress, from any source, stimulates the sympathetic nervous system.

Parasympathetic nervous system activity is restorative, activating the liver, spleen, stomach, intestines, pancreas, kidneys and colon to nourish the body and eliminate toxins. Sauna therapy inhibits sympathetic activity, helping to balance the autonomic nervous system and enhance the activity of the eliminative organs.

To obtain the best detoxification results, the body must be as parasympathetic or relaxed as possible because detoxification requires parasympathetic activity. More rest, a careful diet and other relaxing healing modalities are excellent in conjunction with sauna therapy. I do not recommend exercise before sauna use, although the Hubbard detoxification programs do use exercise to help dislodge toxins. This is an area for future research.

Relieving Internal Congestion

Excessive sympathetic nervous stimulation causes blood to stagnate in the internal organs, impairing normal detoxification. Saunas powerfully shunt blood to the body surface, relieving congestion of the internal organs and assisting their functioning.

Normalizing Alkalinity

Some people's tissues tend to be overly alkaline. Others tend to be excessively acidic. The heat of the sauna increases enzymatic activity that helps balance the pH of the body, helping to dissolve calcium and other chemical deposits.

Enhancing Oxygenation

Impaired oxygenation of the tissues interferes with normal detoxification mechanisms that involve oxidation reactions. Sauna therapy enhances oxygenation of the tissues by shunting blood to the skin and enhancing circulation to the lungs as well. Heating the body also increases the heart rate and blood flow throughout the body, assisting oxygenation.

Deep Tissue Penetration

Heating the tissues from the inside that occurs with infrared lamp saunas and far infrared saunas facilitates detoxification at deeper tissue levels.

Other Infrared Benefits

Infrared energy, of which there is a wider spectrum in the infrared lamp sauna, is itself a nutrient and antioxidant. It facilitates cellular processes, assisting energy production and normal detoxification mechanisms. Infrared also helps decouple toxins from water molecules. This not only assists the elimination of toxins. It also reduces the surface tension of the water in the body to improve hydration and oxygenation of the tissues.

A More Comprehensive Detoxification Program

The above illustrates how sauna therapy can help with detoxification. Even better is to integrate its use with a more complete detoxification program. Here are other methods that are used in nutritional balancing science along with sauna therapy to enhance a detoxification regimen.

1. Reduce Exposure. This means adopting a natural lifestyle and a clean diet, drinking spring water (even in plastic bottles), breathing clean air and avoiding toxic products in the home, office and elsewhere. Other ways to reduce toxin exposure are removing dental amalgams, removing breast implants, and using less toxic cleaners and body care products.

2. Rest More And Reduce Damaging Stress. Detoxification requires energy. Reducing all strenuous activities, including too much exercise, and getting at least nine hours of sleep per night are most helpful for detoxification. Reducing unnecessary activities that deplete energy, simplifying one's life and avoiding fear, worry, anger, guilt and resentments also rest the nervous system.

3. Enhance The Production Of Energy. Elimination of toxins is a body function that requires adequate adaptive energy. *Low energy is often the most important stumbling block to detoxification, especially for slow oxidizers.*

Any substance, therapy or procedure that enhances the body's energy production will assist the elimination of toxins. Lifestyle changes might include improving the diet, more rest, quitting stimulants such as caffeine and sugar, and deep breathing. Eliminating toxic substances from the environment, treating chronic infections and oxygen therapies also help.

Nutrients involved in energy production include many minerals such as copper, iron, zinc, magnesium and manganese among others. Other nutrients required for energy production include coenzyme Q-10 and many vitamins such as B-complex, C, E and others. These are best obtained from the diet. However, supplements may be needed, especially vital minerals that are deficient in today's modern refined foods. Infrared energy is, in fact, a nutrient, as well, that functions as an antioxidant and in other ways.

The Twin Aspects Of Energy Production. There are at least two basic aspects of increasing energy production, 1) *restoring the energy pathways* and 2) *balancing the oxidation rate.* These are analogous to 1) replacing worn parts of an engine and 2) tuning the engine or adjusting its speed for optimum power output.

The energy pathway includes all the steps involved in the production and utilization of energy. This begins with the food one eats, its digestion, and the absorption of nutrients. The pathway also includes the metabolism of nutrients in the liver, transport of nutrients to the cells, and their final utilization in the Krebs and glycolysis energy cycles to produce ATP (adenosine triphosphate). Toxins, infections, nutrient deficiencies, glandular imbalances and other factors can block any of these critical steps in the energy pathway.

Balancing the oxidation rate is often overlooked, but very critical. It enhances energy *efficiency,* much like running an engine at the optimal RPM. All enzymes have an optimal rate and temperature, for example, at which their efficiency is greatest. Many times the best detoxification products and procedures are less effective because energy efficiency is very low. This is like having a great bicycle, but pedaling it in the wrong gear. Hair mineral analysis from a laboratory that does not wash the hair can assess the oxidation rate and guide its correction with diet and nutritional supplements. Sauna therapy also often enhances energy efficiency by helping to balance body chemistry.

4. Enhance Parasympathetic Nervous System Activity. Detoxification is a parasympathetic activity. It involves the liver, kidneys and bowel, all of which are innervated by parasympathetic nerve fibers. Any therapy that promotes parasympathetic activity or inhibits sympathetic activity will assist detoxification. These include:

- Near infrared lamp sauna sessions and coffee enemas.
- Supplements such as pancreatic enzymes, calcium, magnesium, zinc, TMG or trimethylglycine, kelp and a few others, but not most supplements.
- Meditation and relaxation therapies.
- A diet of mainly cooked food, no smoothies, no fruit, and free of stimulants and excitotoxins such as MSG and Aspartame.
- Removing toxic metals and chemicals is extremely helpful. These can keep a body in a sympathetic state.
- Anti-anxiety herbs and other remedies may also be helpful, but often are somewhat toxic so I rarely use them.

5. Assist The Eliminative Organs. The major eliminative organs include the liver, kidneys, lungs, bowel and skin. I use foods and supplements to assist these organs. Saunas are fabulous for the skin and for circulation. Coffee enemas are excellent for the liver and bowels. Deep breathing is most helpful for the lungs and for oxygenation. Kidney glandular substance, is excellent for the kidneys.

In addition, each cell must eliminate toxins to function properly. This depends upon many factors such as the condition of the cell membrane and other cell structures. The circulatory and lymphatic systems play indispensable roles to carry away cellular wastes.

The glands must function well to regulate the activity of the eliminative organs. The autonomic nervous system also plays a critical role. The parasympathetic nervous system enhances the activity of the eliminative organs. *Sympathetic dominance*, a common mineral pattern on a properly performed hair mineral test, diminishes the activity of these organs. Balancing the major ratios on a hair mineral test help all of the eliminative organs.

6. Make the body more yang. This is an extremely important aspect of a complete detoxification regimen. Sauna therapy helps, and so does a careful choice of foods, avoiding fruit and most juices. Certain supplements help, while most others are harmful. Even one's thinking either helps or hinders the balance of yin and yang in the body. For much more on this topic, read *Yin and Yang Healing* at ww.drlwilson.com.

7. Supplement With Antagonists. Toxic metals and chemicals often compete with vital substances in the body for absorption and in metabolic processes such as in enzyme binding sites. One may reduce the absorption and effects of toxins with substances that antagonize toxin absorption or metabolism.

For example, calcium, zinc and selenium are helpful for cadmium toxicity. Zinc, manganese, vitamin B6, molybdenum and sulfur are helpful antagonists for copper toxicity. Administering extra choline may help reduce the effects of pesticides that are cholinesterase inhibitors. Toxins often deplete vitamins or interfere with their metabolism. Giving higher

se nutrients can offset some of the effects of these toxins. Antibiotics and antitoxins
sidered antagonists for bacteria or other toxins.

mprove the digestion. This may not seem important, but it is essential. Most
people digestive system is inflamed and many suffer from a "leaky gut" that allows partially
digested proteins and other toxic substances to be absorbed into the body. Poor digestion also
impairs nutrient absorption that is required for proper detoxification.

Correcting the digestion is not easy. It requires a fairly strict diet, and I find that one must
avoid certain foods, all smoothies, most juices, and other substances that easily upset digestion.

9. Methods of detoxification I suggest avoiding.

a) Chelation. Chelators are substances that bind to toxic metals and help remove them.
Unfortunately, both natural and synthetic drug chelators remove vital minerals along with the
toxic ones. All of them also remove toxic metals in an unnatural order, and they do not remove
them deeply enough. For much more information about chelation therapy, read *Chelation* at
www.drlwilson.com.

b) Homeopathy. Sadly, today I find this older method is too yin and therefore not helpful,
even when it produces symptomatic results.

c) Most herbs. These are also toxic and yin today, and not needed. I use a few herbs such
as dandelion, milk thistle, burdock root, Russian black radish, but not many more.

Other Detoxification Topics

Preferred Minerals

Thousands of enzyme systems in the body depend on minerals as catalysts, facilitators or
as part of the enzyme itself. Each enzyme operates best with a *preferred mineral or minerals*
such as zinc or magnesium. However, when the diet is deficient in vital minerals, the body will
absorb and utilize a toxic metal in many enzymes. Copper or cadmium may replace zinc, for
example.

The toxic metal acts like a replacement part in a car when the original part is not available.
The replacement does not function as well as the original, but can keep one going. Enzymes that
contain toxic metals may function at 5-50%, enough to sustain life. As more of these
accumulate, however, enzymatic activity deteriorates until illness occurs.

*Correction of body chemistry involves the replacement of the preferred minerals in enzyme
binding sites.* The diet must contain the vital minerals, the eliminative organs must function
well, energy must be available to effect the replacement and stress must be at a minimum. It
often takes several years or more of following a healthful regimen, along with the use of
therapies that enhance the process, to restore the preferred minerals in hundreds of thousands of
enzyme binding sites.

Health maintenance and disease prevention involve making sure one obtains all the vital
minerals the body needs. This is difficult today due to hybrid crops low in minerals, refined food
diets, poor eating habits, impaired digestion, contaminated food and water, and stress that
depletes nutrients and hinders digestion.

Most children today are born mineral-deficient due to deficiencies in the parents. Prenatal care needs to begin several years before one becomes pregnant. It takes that long to replenish 20 to 30 minerals and other nutrients. Until these preventive measures are instituted, I fear that toxic metal accumulation and its health effects will become even more common.

Layered Toxins

Toxins are 'layered' within the body. This does not mean they are stacked one on top of each other. However, they are at various cellular levels, with some much more deeply buried than others.

For example, in my experience, one never simply has mercury or lead toxicity. Most of the time, one has mercury beneath some lead, which is beneath copper mixed with pesticides and a chronic infection secreting toxins beneath that. Each layer of toxicity is deeper within organs or other tissues.

Layering means that several years or more may be required for thorough detoxification. One never knows at which layer a toxin is concentrated except by slowly working though the layers. One cannot, for example, eliminate all the lead in the body within six months, although one can eliminate some.

Many physicians run tests looking for a toxic metal or chemical, the removal of which will cure the patient. Tests can be useful, and I am delighted physicians are beginning to become aware of the role of toxic metals and chemicals. However, of much greater importance, in my experience, is designing a program that balances body chemistry while assisting *all* toxin elimination.

Everyone has many toxic metals and chemicals, often present from birth. Also, most people have six to twelve or more chronic infections affecting their health. The advantage of sauna therapy is its effectiveness with all these toxic conditions.

Sauna therapy assists normal detoxification mechanisms rather than forcing out any one toxin. In so doing, *it respects the body's wisdom and the natural order of detoxification of layered toxins.* This approach may seem slower, but is far safer and does much more to improve general health than focusing on just one or a few toxins.

To Detoxify, Remove The Need For Compensations

Many toxins act as compensatory mechanisms. They can boost adrenal and perhaps thyroid activity when the glands are nutritionally depleted, or when one is fatigued or stressed. Toxins will re-accumulate if one simply chelates them or removes them by other means without addressing deeper issues such as nutritional depletion, stress, fatigue and sympathetic nervous system dominance.

Among minerals that act as compensations, cadmium is described as having "an aldosterone-like effect". This means that it mimics the effects of the adrenal hormone, aldosterone, raising the sodium level. This is a very critical compensatory mechanism. Nickel, aluminum, lead, iron, copper and manganese may also compensate for weak adrenal activity. Some organic chemical compounds also act in this compensatory fashion. This is a complex topic involving the balance of body chemistry.

By adding heat and light energy to the body and inhibiting the sympathetic nervous system, saunas can reduce the need for compensatory toxins and produce more permanent detoxification.

Order of Organ Cleanout

The first organs to be assisted by sauna therapy are organs of elimination, notably the skin and then the liver and kidneys. This is an important therapeutic aspect of sauna therapy. By first assisting the organs of elimination, sauna therapy, when done properly, is less prone to the problem of re-depositing toxic metals and chemicals in vital organs.

Toxins Versus Genetics

Today the news often reports that a defective gene is the possible cause for many health conditions. However, we rarely hear the true statement that *toxins, along with nutritional deficiencies, cause defective genetic expression.*

Illness is more often due to defective genetic expression, sometimes called a *polymorphism* in the field of genetics. This fact helps explain why at times those with a genetic disorder such as Down's syndrome are helped dramatically by nutritional and other natural therapies. It is also why young women would be wise to undergo a detoxification program before becoming pregnant to help prevent birth defects in their children.

The Concept of Density

When the body harbors excessive toxic metals and chemicals it actually is more dense. Healing generally involves replacing heavy metals with lighter elements, although some light elements such as aluminum are toxic. Also, healing requires that complex chemicals be broken down into simpler compounds and eliminated through the liver and kidneys.

The concept of reducing the body's density is a primary goal in some practices of yoga, tai chi and chi kung. One learns movements and breathing exercises to open channels to enhance the flow of chi or subtle energy throughout the body. Other natural healing arts embrace similar concepts including acupuncture, acupressure, reiki, chiropractic and some forms of massage.

Sauna therapy is very helpful for reducing the density of the physical body. Improving blood and lymph circulation reduces congestion of the internal organs, rendering them less dense as well. Chapter 2 mentions that infrared radiation can decouple toxins from water molecules. This, too, may help reduce excessive density.

Benefits include reduced sensitivity to microwaves, radio frequency and other electrical fields, and perhaps improvement in 'magnetic deficiency syndrome', which can be associated with iron and/or manganese imbalance. Mineral analysis reveals that iron and manganese toxicity are quite common. Other benefits of reducing density include enhanced personality and spiritual development, improved awareness, better relationships and overall better health.

Healing Facility Or Home Therapy

Sauna detoxification can occur at a health facility or in one's home. Health facilities offer close supervision. Programs are often more intense and for this reason the results can be more rapid. Many residential programs use the Hubbard protocol and involve spending several hours daily in a traditional hot air sauna for several weeks or more. Control over a person's diet and physical activity is easier at a facility. Away from family, work and friends, healing may progress faster. A clinic program also provides structure and discipline that some people require.

Disadvantages of health facilities are their cost and, if in a distant city, the need to take several weeks away from family and work. Also, several weeks of treatment will improve many conditions but may not be enough to correct deep-seated illnesses and deeper layers of toxicity.

Home-based Therapy

Therapy at home costs less and one need not leave work or family. Children and the disabled can participate more easily and the program can continue for months or longer. Sauna sessions are 20-60 minutes in the morning and/or evening, allowing a fairly normal lifestyle. Discipline is required, however, and one must have daily access to a sauna.

Results will be somewhat slower at home because one spends less time in treatment. As a result, however, healing reactions are also less severe. Close supervision is less necessary than with more intense programs.

Most people can do home sauna therapy, including children five and older and many who are ill or elderly. Those with diagnosed health conditions should inform their doctor and may need special instructions. Frail or elderly persons should begin with only 15 minutes in the sauna, preferably with an aide or attendant standing by. One who is terminally ill may use a sauna for symptom relief and perhaps life extension.

One can also combine home therapy with periodic treatment at a health facility. This book is designed mainly for home-based therapy.

Potential Detoxification Program Difficulties

1. Improper procedures. A detoxification program will be much less effective if it is not intense enough, too intense, improperly combined with other therapies or poorly monitored. Extremely important, for example, is getting enough rest.

2. Lack of supervision. Throughout any sauna detoxification program, supervision and support are important. Insisting on supervision and feedback is the responsibility of both the supervising practitioner and the client.

3. Confusing illness with the healing effects of the sauna. Repeated heating of the body causes physiological changes that can easily be mistaken for illness. Symptoms may include rashes, headaches, flare-ups of chronic infections and more. Most of these symptoms are benign and pass quickly. Some, however, may be acute and vigorous, and occasionally may take several weeks to resolve. This topic is covered in more detail in Chapter 11, Healing Reactions.

4. Toxin redistribution. To be eliminated, toxins must first be removed from their storage sites in the body. They must move into the bloodstream or into the lymph system. From here, they move to the liver, kidneys, bowel, lungs or skin for elimination. It is possible that during this process, some toxins could redeposit somewhere in the body. This is a concern with any method or system of detoxification.

My experience is with several thousand people of all ages who follow a nutritional balancing program that includes daily use of a near infrared lamp sauna. When sauna therapy is employed in this manner, toxin redistribution does not occur to any sizable degree. I have not heard of significant toxin redistribution with other sauna programs, but theoretically it could occur. This is one of the main reasons I always suggest following a complete healing program when doing sauna therapy.

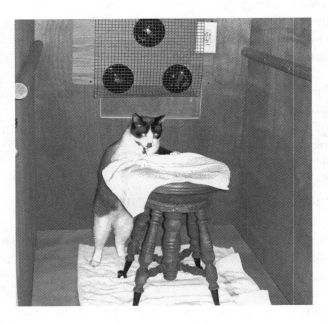

"Will someone turn on the lights?"

6
Other Aspects Of Sauna Therapy

I have had severe pain and pressure over my left eye and radiating down the left side of my face for three years. No doctor has been able to help. After only two months of using an infrared lamp sauna, the pressure is gone.

After four days of the sauna therapy, I awoke with a very sore throat and head congestion. In a week, that went away and I started having a foul-smelling yellowy mucus discharge from my nose. That lasted about a week. Then I developed a terrible headache that required Excedrin for the pain. I still get headaches at times, so I am continuing with sauna therapy. I set up an infrared lamp sauna in my small bathroom and I use it one hour per day (two half-hour sessions). - Mrs. S. S., Chads Ford, PA.

Some other healing modalities can enhance the benefits of sauna sessions. Others that are in common use are toxic and should be avoided. This chapter discusses the use of meditation, visualization, sound, music, breathing, oxygen, negative ions, light, color, niacin, charcoal, other vitamins or minerals, massage, exercise, posture, steam and aromatherapy during sauna sessions.

Meditation

The Roy Masters Judeo-Christian meditation is a fabulous addition to sauna therapy. It is one of the most amazing exercises one can do one's whole life. I highly recommend it. This is the only meditation I am able to recommend because it is the only one that moves energy firmly downward through the body. All others may be harmful, and are not recommended, including almost all Western and Eastern types. They do not move energy straight downward, and this is their problem. For more on this subject, read the article, *Meditation* at **www.drlwilson.com**.

Visualization

Visualization brings the mind into play in a different way than the Roy Masters meditation described above. It can help you relax in a sauna and may help overcome mental resistance to new experiences that can occur during sauna therapy. Here are several visualization exercises:

1) An excellent exercise is to imagine, as one inhales, that one is absorbing warmth and red light from the sauna. Imagine one is pulling this energy into the body and, at the same time,

downward from the head, down the front of the body. Visualize the energy moving from the head down into the fingers and toes. As one exhales, continue the process. As any angry, resentful or otherwise negative thoughts arise, imagine letting them go as one 'sweats them out'. This visualization can enhance the ability to absorb color and infrared energy. Deep, slow, relaxed breathing is best. Do not strain or force anything. With practice, one may feel as though every cell in the body breathes. This is powerful and similar to the Roy Masters Judeo-Christian exercise mentioned above.

A variant is that on the exhale of the breath, see and even feel the energy turn around and flow up the back or spine, (not the front of the body), arriving finally at the top of the head. Then, as you inhale again, the energy turns around and begins flowing down the front of the body. This is called *circle breathing* or the *microcosmic orbit* in some older texts. It is a very powerful way to clear blocked energy in the body.

2) Pick your favorite prayer such as the 23Psalm of David in the bible, or another if you prefer. Focus on it while absorbing the sauna's healing energy. This can help teach simple concentration and focus, and helps you relax.

3) Just relax and let the mind drift. This is fine for beginners to increase enjoyment of the sauna. However, using the mind to meditate or visualize while in the sauna offers much greater possibilities for healing.

Aromatherapy

I do not recommend aromatherapy, in general, because it is too yin and always somewhat toxic. The heat of a sauna may enhance the effects of aromatherapy, so please be careful. Aromatherapy is not needed during a nutritional balancing program.

Do not place oils of any kind on the skin just before a sauna session in a location where infrared light may reach them. The oils could heat up excessively and cause a burn.

Sound

Sound is another ancient, effective healing modality that is simple to incorporate into a sauna session. It may be music, chanting or tones from a piano, synthesizer or other instrument.

Relaxing music can reduce sympathetic nervous system activity if one is tense when entering a sauna. Relaxation greatly facilitates detoxification. Listening to soothing music is excellent for beginners. More powerful effects will accrue from using specific tones or frequencies. Low tones from a piano or low chanting tones are excellent to break up congestion of the internal organs and other tissues.

To experience this, place a speaker or portable stereo on top or inside of the sauna to play tapes or CDs. Buy a compact disc of low chanting, or I currently offer a CD of these tones played on a piano. Alternatively, make your own recording.

Conscious Breathing

Many people breathe in a shallow way. Some also hold their breath too long or do not fill all regions of their lungs. These habits can contribute to physical and emotional imbalances.

They may also cause breathing difficulties during a sauna session. Sitting in a sauna offers an excellent opportunity to correct one's breathing habits, filling the lungs and moving the diaphragm in a slow and rhythmic fashion.

Deep breathing massages the internal organs in a way no other method can. It enhances blood circulation, assists lymphatic drainage, helps eliminate toxins, helps oxygenate the tissues and relieves congestion and stagnation in the organs. Slow, relaxed, deep breathing also reduces the activity of the sympathetic nervous system. This is very relaxing and enhances the detoxifying effects of the sauna.

An excellent and ancient breathing pattern for healing mind and body is the three-part yoga breath. During the first part, inhale into the abdomen, pushing the abdomen outward. Then fill the mid-chest and allow it to expand out to the sides. Finally, fill the upper chest with air. Your chest should rise in front. Exhale from the chest down.

Do this in a smooth rhythm, slowly counting to nine. Allow three counts as you fill each of the three parts of your chest. Hold your breath in for a count of three if possible. Then exhale also to a count of nine. Counting helps maintain an even breathing rhythm.

Toe Breathing. This is another superb breathing exercise. As you inhale, imagine the air entering the body through the toes, and remaining in the feet. Hold your breath for a count of about three or four seconds, and then exhale through the feet and toes. The purpose of this exercise is to keep your mind focused downward at your feet. This will help keep moving subtle energy downward, which is excellent for one's health and development.

Another exercise is to visualize your body cavity as a large vase. On the inhale, it fills with water. On the exhale, you open a drain plug and the water slowly pours out.

Breathing Difficulties. Saunas are usually well tolerated by those with lung, bronchial or sinus problems. Warm air dilates the bronchial tubes and nasal passages, and helps drain the sinuses. Steam vapor helps some, but for others the heat and steam can make breathing difficult. Those with emphysema or other serious respiratory problems should begin with less time in a sauna and notice how well they tolerate it.

If there is difficulty breathing in a full-body sauna, open the door slightly to allow fresh, cool air to enter and to allow odors and toxic gases to escape. If breathing is still difficult, an alternative is to breathe through a one-inch flexible plastic tube connected to outside air through a ventilation opening. Rarely, those with severe breathing problems may require a sauna cabinet with the head outside the sauna exposed to fresh air.

Posture

Improper or poor posture can be an important contributor to physical ailments as it can impair breathing, reduce oxygenation of vital organs, and even cause muscle strain and spinal subluxations. Posture also has much to do with self-esteem and self-image, which can be important for healing. The sauna is an excellent place to practice proper posture and alignment of the body.

Sit comfortably in a sauna. Avoid slouching and leaning as much as possible. This will enhance the effects of the session and prevent back strain and muscular tension. While sitting, imagine a string attached to the crown of the head. This is not the top of the head, but slightly toward the back of the head. Imagine someone pulling up on this string, gently drawing the head upward, away from the body and extending the neck. The head does not tilt forward or back. It remains level with the eyes looking straight ahead.

At the same time, relax the rest of the body. Let the shoulders and arms droop, and let the chest and back relax. Imagine that the string at the crown of your head holds up the entire body as you relax. Much tension is often held in the shoulders. They should round slightly as they relax. Many people also puff up the chest and back without realizing it. These should relax and flatten as one relaxes. Doing slow neck rolls while in the sauna is also very relaxing.

Also practice gently rocking the pelvis back and forth in a rhythmic way. In many people, the pelvis is locked in one position, often tilted backward. This places tension on the low back and can impair circulation to the pelvic area. Allow the pelvis to move and practice until it moves freely.

With practice, one can combine gentle rocking of the pelvis with rhythmic breathing. Inhaling into the abdomen, the pelvis should tilt slightly forward. On the exhale, the pelvis tilts slightly backward. Eventually, the low back should relax and the pelvis should sit comfortably directly under your head. The ear, shoulder and hipbones should be underneath one another in a straight line.

Eye Exercises

A few minutes of eye exercises can also be easily incorporated into a sauna session. These can be as simple as looking up on an the inhale and down on the exhale. Then do the same looking left and right, followed by the same in diagonals and then move the eyes in a circle. One can also coordinate the exercises with deep breathing and focusing on healing intentions.

Color

Colors impact specific organs, body systems and chakras or energy centers. Color therapy is a powerful healing modality and a logical adjunct to sauna therapy. The near infrared lamp sauna offers built-in color therapy that is best for most people. It provides red, orange and yellow light that moves energy downward to the lower chakras that are often most in need of healing. Other colored lights can be added to a sauna, but I don't usually recommend them as they are not needed and interfere with energy moving downward through the body.

Color therapy researcher Dinshaw Ghadiali found that red stimulates the adrenals, testes, ovaries and growth. Red also clears the emotional body, helping to eliminate emotional toxins. Note, however, there is a difference between *red* and the *infrared* produced by the lamp sauna. This was brought to light by Ms. Luwanna Rine, a color therapist. She shined a red lamp on dogs, and made them more irritable. However, when she shined a red infrared heat lamp on the same animals, they calmed down and their health improved.

In the classical color therapy literature, orange stimulates the intestines, liver, pancreas and assimilation. Yellow stimulates the stomach, spleen and digestion. As many of these organs assist elimination, exposure to these colors in conjunction with the sauna's heat may significantly enhance the detoxifying and healing effects of sauna therapy.

Green is balancing for the nervous system and very healing. Blue, indigo and violet are cooling. They also activate the thyroid, pituitary and pineal glands. Cooling energy may not be helpful in a sauna, which is a heating experience, ideally. It may help in a few cases.

Exercise

L. Ron Hubbard believed patients should exercise with a stationary bike before entering a sauna. The concept was to enhance circulation and thus enhance detoxification. Sauna detoxification programs modeled on the Hubbard regimen continue this recommendation.

However, exercise requires expending energy that could be conserved for healing. Also, exercise activates the sympathetic nervous system. This definitely interferes with detoxification. For these reasons, do not exercise before entering a sauna. Mild exercise is beneficial, however, as part of a total health program. This is discussed in the chapter that follows.

Reflexology And Massage

Reflexology is a very safe and powerful healing method. It is also easy to use. Before, during, or after your sauna sessions, press firmly all over each foot and/or each hand. Include the toes and fingers, and the tops and bottoms of the feet and hands. This has a strong relaxing, balancing and detoxifying effect on the entire body. Maps of the reflexology points are available at no charge on the internet. Also, to release tension, "pop" the toes by pushing them down.

A short massage before or after a sauna session is fine to help one relax, improve circulation and perhaps release more toxins. *However, professional massage is not safe, especially for young women.*

Water

Drink about 8-16 ounces of quality spring water, ideally, before and after using a sauna. Drinking water while in the sauna is fine, but will diminish the intensity of the sauna effect a little bit. If you do not have spring water, tap water *filtered with only carbon* is second best, in many cases. Other filters such as KDF and other media damage tap water and are not suggested at all. Also, *do not drink reverse osmosis water, alkaline waters, water with salt, or most other types of water.* These can be very harmful. For more on water, see *Chapter 7* or read **Water For Drinking** at **www.drlwilson.com.**

Steam

Steam is often part of the experience in traditional saunas and Native American sweat lodges. One splashes water on hot rocks to produce the steam. Steam is at 212° F. As it circulates, it releases its heat when condensing on the bather's skin or other surfaces in the sauna.

This adds a lot of heat very quickly. The sauna may also feel hotter because the added humidity reduces sweating somewhat. Adding steam can make a sauna feel much hotter.

The advantages of steam for some people are the higher temperature and higher humidity plus the conductive effect of the steam on the skin. The effect is called "loyli" in Finnish sauna lore. Some people breathe more easily and deeper with steam, and feel more relaxed as well.

However, adding steam can quickly increase the sauna's temperature to 200° F. or above. This interferes with healing, and perhaps even with breathing. Steam is not a part of near infrared sauna therapy, and is not recommended or needed.

Ozone

Oxygen or ozone can be pumped into a sauna. This can facilitate oxygenation of the tissues and detoxification of the body. Especially for those living in urban areas with a low oxygen content, adding oxygen or ozone can be superb.

Ozone is O3, a less stable form of oxygen. Once inside the body, it releases extra oxygen atoms. Ozone is perfectly safe when used correctly, although too much can irritate the lungs when inhaled. This is the only reason it is considered an air pollutant.

Oxygen is non-irritating and also easily pumped in to any sauna. Two types of oxygen are available. One is pure oxygen in a tank. This is widely used in hospitals, but is somewhat unwieldy as the tanks are heavy and a bit costly. The other method is an oxygen concentrator. This is a device that separates the oxygen and nitrogen in the air and discards the nitrogen so that oxygen is concentrated. These units are still costly, but can be purchased or rented.

While it can be added to a sauna, a much better way to obtain more oxygen is to install an ozonator/ionizer air purifier in your bedroom. At this time, I suggest the machine sold by Better Living Alpine Air at **www.betterlivingalipineair.com** or a similar unit.

Ozone can also be taken in your water or even intravenously, administered by a skilled physician. For more information about intravenous ozone, contact the International Oxidative Medicine Association (800-235-4788) or the International Bio-Oxidative Medicine Foundation.

Niacin

In the 1950s, L. Ron Hubbard pioneered the use of niacin in 1000mg to 5000 mg doses daily with sauna therapy, supposedly to open the pores. However, I find it to be definitely toxic. ***Do not use niacin in doses above about 50 mg daily.*** Niacin suppresses peripheral sympathetic nervous system activity. This causes peripheral vasodilation and a prickly sensation of the skin.

Cool Bathing and Cold Plunges

Extreme cold after a sauna is neither necessary nor recommended. After a sauna session, a warm or tepid shower is best. The shower temperature should be comfortable, not icy cold. Extreme cold causes a sympathetic reaction that may slow or stop detoxification.

Charcoal Tablets

Charcoal is an excellent material to absorb many toxins from the intestines. However, charcoal also absorbs nutrient minerals from the intestines and causes their removal from the body. For this reason, I do not suggest charcoal tablets, except perhaps for diarrhea or another severe healing reaction, and then only for a few hours or a day or two at most.

A Full Spectrum Bulb To Supply Vitamin D

A sauna is an excellent place to expose the body to full-spectrum light if you are unclothed or wearing just a skimpy bathing suit in the sauna, which is fine to do. Adding a full-spectrum bulb to a sauna will slightly increase vitamin D production. However, newer research indicates that it is not helpful to supply enough vitamin D for most people.

If you wish to add a light bulb for vitamin D, it only works if you expose *the middle of the chest* to quite intense ultraviolet radiation (UVB). This method of obtaining vitamin D is unreliable and I suggest all adults take about 5000 iu daily of vitamin D3, or take vitamin D2 if you do not tolerate vitamin D3 for some reason. An excellent alternative is to eat 3-4 cans of sardines weekly and this should supply enough vitamin D.

There is a growing consensus that more vitamin D is needed by everyone, especially in the winter months, regardless of where you live or how much you are out in the sun. Those with dark skin or those living above 40 degrees latitude (Around Reno, Nevada; Denver, Colorado; Indianapolis, Indiana; or Philadelphia, Pennsylvania) need even more vitamin D. This vitamin performs many crucial roles in the body. These include calcium absorption, genetic regulation and regulation of normal cell division. It is also involved in immune function, insulin secretion, blood clotting and blood pressure control.

In a meta-analysis by C.F. Garland et al. published in the February 2006 issue of the *American Journal of Public Health*, the authors reviewed 63 studies of vitamin D status and cancer risk. They found that a majority of the studies showed a protective role for vitamin D.

To slightly enhance vitamin D production, add one or more 100-watt or greater full-spectrum light bulbs to your sauna. The least expensive is a GE Reveal bulb. Others are Cromolux or a fluorescent type. Sit with your chest as close as possible to the full-spectrum lamp. If possible, have your chest positioned within several inches of the lamp. The dangers of overdosing on vitamin D are mostly exaggerated. An excessive amount may cause some sleepiness.

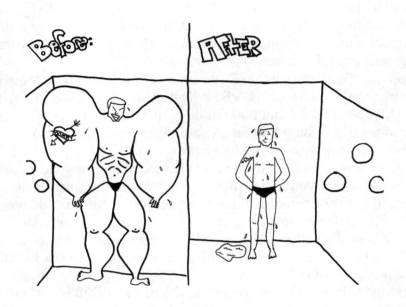

"Joe sweats out the steroids."

7

A More Complete Healing Program

"I have used an infrared lamp sauna daily for two years and have noticed the following: I feel warmer and do not need sweaters in air conditioned restaurants. Blood circulation is better and I obtained relief from chronic nasal congestion. I also have medical tests proving that my liver and kidneys function better.

I have not had a single cold or flu in two years, my skin is supple and I look and feel younger. I am also much more moderate in my emotional responses, which has made life calmer and more balanced.

If I have the chance to build a new house, it will definitely have an infrared lamp sauna in the bathroom, as I believe that sauna therapy has improved my health greatly. I consider it one of the easiest, least expensive and most effective ways to cleanse my lymphatic system and internal organs. - Mrs. T. M., Valrico, FL

Sauna therapy is much more effective and safer when accompanied by a complete healing program. The program needs to include plenty of rest and sleep, a healthful diet, proper drinking water, and a few nutritional supplements. Also helpful are healthy attitudes, emotional control and, when needed, other therapies such as chiropractic. This chapter discusses the basics of such a program. An excellent approach is a complete nutritional balancing program with one of the Approved Practitioners listed at **www.drlwilson.com**.

Diet

A diet for development. The suggestions in this chapter may seem unusual because the goal is *development* of a human being. *Development* is a precise science that promotes health and long life, but is largely unknown today. The details are discussed at **www.drlwilson.com**.

The need for alkaline reserve minerals. The dietary suggestions in this section focus on providing certain minerals that are missing in everyone today. Most of these minerals cannot be obtained from pills, but only from a diet rich in *cooked, not raw* vegetables. Other ways to obtain them are to use sea salt, bone broth, and drinking water such as spring water or tap water. Do not use reverse osmosis water or distilled water, which are very low in minerals.

What To Eat. *Protein.* This is critical for liver detoxification and to rebuild the body. The best ones are:

Lamb – an excellent food. (Eat red meat only twice per week).

Wild game – also very good, except avoid buffalo and bison, which do not work as well.

Chicken – especially dark meat chicken. Very good and may be eaten daily.

Sardines – the best fish. They are very low in mercury due to their size. 3-4 standard-sized cans weekly provide many nutrients. *Avoid all other fish*, because they are too high in mercury.

Toasted almond butter – also excellent as a daily food.

Eggs – good, but women should have up to 6 eggs per week only. Men may have up to 8 eggs per week. Cook eggs so the yolks are runny, either soft-boiled for 3 minutes, poached or lightly fried. *Avoid* hard-cooked eggs.

Duck and turkey - also good once or twice weekly.

Cheese, yogurt, kefir – not as good for development, but you may have a total of four ounces daily (about 110 ml) of all of the dairy proteins combined. Raw or organic are best. Do not cook cheese.

Lentils, split peas or other beans. These are not quite as good. Have them up to twice weekly.

Beef, tofu, tempeh – not quite as good. Skip them or have them at most once or twice weekly.

Other rules. Limit animal protein to twice daily. Avoid vegetarian and vegan diets because they are deficient diets. Limit portions of protein foods to 4-5 ounces (110-150 ml) each. Avoid *all* protein powders, smoothies and shakes. Whole foods are much better for development.

Avoid pork, ham, lard and bacon as they often contain parasite cysts, even if well-cooked. Avoid processed meats such as hot dogs, bologna and salami, as these usually contain many additives. Also *avoid* food bars (bad combinations) and refined soy protein. Except for toasted almond butter, avoid nuts and seeds. They are nutritious, but a little toxic and harder to digest.

Vegetables. Lots of cooked vegetables are needed today. Do not skip them! The best are:

Roots: all onions, scallions, shallots, leaks, pearl onions, carrots, rutabaga, and daikon radish. Eat the others sparingly such as sweet potato, yam, turnips, beets, celery root, parsnip and others.

Cruciferous vegetables: Brussels sprouts, red cabbage, cauliflower (all colors), baby broccoli.

Greens and others: green beans, green onions, and cauliflower leaves are also excellent.

Eat sparingly: other greens, celery, okra, peas, artichoke hearts, and asparagus.

Avoid the nightshade vegetables: potato, tomato, eggplant, and peppers (hot and sweet ones).

Other rules: Fresh is best. Cook all vegetables. Ideally use a pressure-cooker. Crock pots or steaming are the next best methods of cooking. Eat at least 5 different vegetables with each meal. Eat **2-3 cups (450-650 ml) of cooked vegetables with each meal**. Cook vegetables because: 1) cooking breaks down tough vegetable fibers, allowing the body to absorb many more minerals and other phytonutrients, 2) proper cooking makes vegetables much more yang, 3) cooking reduces the volume of the vegetables so that one can eat more of them.

Most people do not eat nearly enough cooked vegetables. Add flavor with herbs, or add a little butter or grated raw cheese, yogurt or cream on top as a dressing. Organically grown vegetables are better.

Grains. These are good for development. Eat about 0.5-1.5 cups (100-350 ml) daily.

Blue corn is excellent for development, even in the form of organic blue corn tortilla chips. These contain a little vegetable oil. However, the oil preserves the corn and is okay to eat. Some people can tolerate blue corn only if it is eaten alone. This problem tends to go away if one follows a nutritional balancing program.

Other acceptable grains are **old-fashioned oats, rye, barley, kamut, amaranth, quinoa,** or noodles made of corn or quinoa. Rice products contain a little arsenic, so they are less recommended at this time (2017). We hope this will be stopped very soon. Cold cereals are not as good. Fast oxidizers can add a little butter to cereal. Do not add fruit or sweeteners to cereal.

Avoid All Wheat and spelt. Years of hybridization have made wheat an irritant to the digestive tract. Especially avoid all white flour, also called *wheat flour*. It has been stripped of nutrients, bleached and altered in other harmful ways.

Some people must eliminate all gluten-containing grains. They must avoid wheat, rye, barley, kamut, spelt and oats. One needs to read labels.

Fats and Oils. These are essential for good health. The best ones are:

Butter and cream. Ghee is also okay, but not quite as good as butter because it is heated.

Meat fat, such as the fat on dark-meat chicken, duck, lamb, and wild game.

Fat from soft-cooked eggs is an excellent fat. Never eat hard-cooked eggs.

Fat in almond butter. Occasionally one can have some other nut butters, but they are all somewhat difficult to digest.

Olive oil. Some is okay. Vary your fats and do not just have olive oil.

Vegetable oils such as corn, peanut, soy and others can be used in moderation.

Nut and seed oils. These are more yin, but a little is okay such as sesame, sunflower, safflower and macadamia nut oils.

Avoid tropical fruit oils, which are very yin. These are coconut oil and all coconut products, palm oil and avocado. Cottonseed oil is heavily sprayed and best avoided.   Avoid French fries, all deep-fried foods, margarine and shortening.

Rules. Fast oxidizers need to add about 3 tablespoons of fat daily to their food. Slow oxidizers need not add extra fat beyond what is in their food. Cream is very good for babies and children.

Avoid Simple Carbohydrates. These include all fruits, fruit juices and all sugary foods. Fruit upsets blood sugar and accumulates a toxic potassium compound from N-P-K fertilizers. Also avoid soy milk, rice milk, almond milk, hemp milk, ice cream, coconut water or milk, and other sweet foods. Adults may have a little goat or cows milk, preferably raw or organic.

Avoid candy, cookies, cakes, pastries, ice cream and soda pop. These cause wide fluctuations in blood sugar and insulin levels. Do not substitute aspartame (Nutrasweet or Equal), saccharin, Splenda or other artificial sweeteners. If you must use a sweetener, xylitol or stevia are best. *Avoid* all prepared foods that contain sugar, honey, maple syrup, dextrose, glucose, fructose, corn syrup, rice bran syrup, chocolate or malt sweetener.

Food combining. A simple rule is to have about 70% cooked vegetables with each meal. In addition, have either **one** type of starch OR **one** type of protein. Keeping food combinations simple greatly eases digestion. Vary your foods, however, by rotating what you eat.

How Much Food. To get enough nutrition, eat three full meals or more daily. Do not skip meals, do not fast, and do not do long cleansing diets. These will worsen your nutritional status.

Condiments.   Good ones are sea salt, mustard, garlic, ginger and other mild herbs and spices. *Avoid* table salt, which is highly refined and low in trace minerals. Table pepper (black pepper) is often rancid, toxic and best avoided. It may also contribute to joint pain and other problems as it is a member of the nightshade family.

Snacks. Ideally, do not snack. If needed, eat an extra sit-down meal in mid-morning or mid-afternoon. This is easy if you cook a lot of vegetables in the morning and eat some at every meal. If you must snack, decent snacks are turkey or beef jerky, raw goat cheese, a soft-cooked egg, some blue corn chips, or leftover chicken and vegetables. Do not snack all day.

Cooking and Food Preparation. Pressure-cooking food is best. Drink the water in which the food is cooked. Other good methods are crock pots, steaming and stir-frying. Cook food until it is soft. Humans do not absorb minerals well from raw food. *Avoid* microwaving, deep-frying, and most roasting or baking. These methods do more damage to food.

Cookware can be made of glass, stainless steel, enamel, or aluminum if it is coated. Electric steamers made of plastic are fine. *Avoid* exposed aluminum cookware, and iron and copper cookware. Making the simple effort to nurture yourself by preparing healthy meals is often important for healing and development.

Eating Habits. Eat regular, relaxed, sit-down meals. Eat slowly and consciously, and chew thoroughly. Chewing each mouthful at least ten times will slow eating and improve digestion. Stop eating before you feel stuffed. Sit quietly at least five to ten minutes after eating. Even better, take a short nap after a large meal. Make meals an enjoyable time. Keep the conversation pleasant. If possible, do not criticize family members at meals.

Avoid eating in a car or while standing up, talking on the telephone or rushing around. These habits can seriously impair digestion and reduce the value of your meal.

Meal Suggestions: Have 2-3 cups (450-650 ml) of well-cooked vegetables with each meal. Ideally, have a little of about 5 or 6 different cooked vegetables. With this, have **one** protein OR **one** starch. For example, for protein have a chicken thigh or leg, or 1-2 lamb chops, or a soft-cooked egg. Instead of protein, you could have a non-wheat cereal or blue corn chips. Ideally, eat your protein first, then vegetables, and then grain. *Rotate foods for best nutrition.*

Eating in restaurants. Frequent eating out is not recommended due to the lower quality of a lot of restaurant food. Among the best restaurants are often Chinese, East Indian or Thai. Food is often made fresh, and they usually offer high-quality protein and cooked vegetables. Ask for extra vegetables.

Rules. When eating out, ask for exactly what you want, even if it is not on the menu. Many restaurants will accommodate you. If bread is served, ask that it be taken away.

Avoid all fast-food and most chain restaurants. They often cut corners and use inferior-quality food. They also use more chemical additives and flavor enhancers such as MSG (monosodium glutamate). Mexican food may contain too much carbohydrate. In a Mexican restaurant, ask for corn, not flour tortillas, and ask for vegetables.

Beverages

Healthful minerals found in mineral-rich water are needed by everyone. Each day, all adults need to drink about 3 quarts, 3 liters, or 96 ounces of preferably high-quality spring water or, in the USA, tap water filtered only with carbon or a sand filter. Tap water in some other nations is not safe to drink. If you drink spring water, vary the brands to obtain different minerals.

One cup of coffee and a cup or two of mild herb tea is okay, but no more. 10-12 ounces (350-400 ml) of carrot juice daily, or 1-2 ounces (about 50 ml) of wheat grass juice twice per week are also good.

Avoid reverse osmosis water, as it does not tend to hydrate the body well enough. Also avoid alkaline water above pH 8.5. It is too yin in macrobiotic terms, and often passes over platinum plates that are toxic. *Avoid* soda pop, sugar-free sodas, alcohol, fruit juices, punch and other soft drinks. Avoid green drinks and juices, other than some carrot juice or wheat grass juice. Most juice is extremely yin. Drinking water while in a sauna is all right.

The best diet for development is an ongoing research project. For updates to this diet, visit **www.drlwilson.com**.

Supplementary Nutrients

Recommended Supplements. While on a sauna therapy program, take 9-15 kelp tablets or 3-6 kelp capsules (about 600 mg each), or up to two tablespoons of kelp granules daily. These supplements provide electrolyte replacement and trace minerals. They also assist detoxification.

Also, include at least 1 teaspoon of sea salt in your daily diet. This can be cooked into foods or added after cooking. *Real Salt* by Redmond is a good brand of sea salt.

Bowel Movements And Laxative Supplements. It is vital to keep the bowels moving. Have at least one bowel movement per day. Constipation may occur as certain toxins are eliminated. Drinking 3 liters or 3 quarts of preferably spring water daily, and eating a lot of cooked vegetables each day, solves most constipation problems.

Coffee enemas with sauna therapy are wonderful to help avoid constipation and to help alleviate symptoms of healing reactions that occur with sauna therapy.

Other Products. Supplements needed by most every adult include 5000 iu daily of vitamin D, 900 mg daily of omega-3 fatty acids, and kelp, as mentioned above. However, if you eat 3 cans of sardines daily, do not supplement vitamin D and omega-3 fatty acids because you will get enough in the sardines.

Other basic supplements are 750 mg of calcium and 450 mg of magnesium daily as chelates or citrates, 20 mg of zinc, up to 1000 mg of TMG or trimethylglycine, a digestive aid such as ox bile and pancreatin, and a low-potency multiple vitamin-mineral tablet.

Some physicians recommend other supplements with sauna therapy. I find these are rarely needed, and often unbalance the body. One must exercise extreme care with supplements because all of them are yin in macrobiotic terminology. Most herbs are also more yin and often somewhat toxic. They are best not taken for prolonged periods of time.

Supplements need to be recommended by someone knowledgeable in the use of saunas for detoxification and healing. Random or inappropriate supplementation can impair or even halt the progress of sauna therapy. See **www.drlwilson.com** for a list of recommended practitioners.

Rest

Extra rest is one of the most important aspects of this program. The basic idea is to conserve the body's energy for healing. Also, many people will feel more tired, at times, during a sauna therapy program. This is normal and should not be of concern. Ideally, sleep nine or more hours every night. At times, naps or other rest periods during the day may also be needed. If possible, have some fresh air in the room when sleeping. Extra rest greatly enhances detoxification and healing.

Exercise

Mild exercise, such as slow walking for up to 30 minutes, is acceptable for those who are physically fit. Vigorous exercise is recommended in some detoxification programs to stimulate circulation or for other reasons. However, I do not recommend it. Exercise uses up energy and I find it best to conserve energy for healing. The sauna provides many of the benefits of exercise such as improved circulation and maintaining muscle tone, while requiring the expenditure of much less energy.

At times during sauna therapy you may feel a burst of energy. However, for best results it is best to avoid strenuous and exhausting activities even when your energy level is high.

Healing Attitudes

The mind is much more powerful than one might imagine. Thoughts and attitudes either enhance or impede the healing process. While entire books deal with this topic, here are some basics. A positive outlook and positive emotions deeply felt have major beneficial effects on our bodies. This has been proven many times. Negative thinking and pessimistic attitudes impair healing because they can act as self-fulfilling prophesies.

Taking full responsibility for every situation in one's life is a wonderful attitude that speeds progress on many levels. Insisting on playing the victim - of other people, of one's birth, one's health condition or other circumstances - slows one's progress and may prevent healing altogether. After all, a victim is not supposed to be truly happy and healthy.

Forgiving everyone who has ever harmed you, no matter who it is, and no matter what occurred, is another very helpful attitude. It can take a while, so begin now. An attitude of gratitude for what you have is also most helpful, no matter how ill you feel. Try to do something you enjoy each day. Learn to love others, although this does not mean you must stay near them, and it does not mean to excuse and dismiss their negative behaviors.

To help cultivate these attitudes, I strongly recommend the Roy Masters Judeo-Christian meditation exercise. For much more information about it, please read Meditation For Healing at www.drlwilson.com.

Healthful Relationships

We are all affected by the energy of others around us. Compatibility in relationships is an important subject, and one to take seriously. *Being tied to unhealthy relationships is a major cause of illness.* Carefully evaluate all of your relationships, including family, friends, business associates, mates and co-workers. Methods of evaluation include meditation, prayers, reading some books, and perhaps counseling.

Do your best to become aware as to whether your relationships are serving your good, and whether they are serving the highest good of all involved. Many relationships are harmful, but the people involved do not realize it. For example, taking responsibility for others when they should be doing this for themselves, is not health-producing for you or for the other person in most cases, even if it appears differently.

This does not mean that relationships will always be easy. However, they should not be destructive. Rest assured, as you consciously choose to serve a greater good, you will attract new friends, new co-workers or job situations, and new, better partners as well.

Colon Cleansing

Colon cleansing using 1 to 4 coffee enemas each day is a superb detoxification method that is fully compatible with near infrared sauna therapy, as recommended in this book. For the procedure I suggest, and much more about them, read **Coffee Enemas** at **www.drlwilson.com.**

Meditation

Meditating daily using the Roy Masters exercise is a wonderful addition to any sauna therapy program. I do not recommend any other type of meditation, as this is the only one I have found that sends energy directly downward from the head to the feet, and this is safest and best. For more on meditation, read the **Meditation** article at **www.drlwilson.com.**

Other Natural Therapies

Many natural therapies can help remove blockages and imbalances, improve subtle energies, and otherwise strengthen the body. Knowledgeable practitioners should familiarize themselves with the benefits of colon cleansing, chiropractic and osteopathic manipulation. Foot reflexology, acupuncture, bodywork, quality massage and other superb therapies can also balance and assist healing of the body.

Clothing, Breathing and Negative Thoughts

Wear loose-fitting, natural fiber clothing at all times to help preserve and assist skin circulation. In a sauna, preferably do not wear much clothing, although a skimpy bathing suit is fine.

If possible, breathe fresh air at all times. Breathe deeply and slowly. This is very relaxing for the nervous system and an excellent meditative practice to do all day. Work on letting go of all negative thoughts. Unusual thoughts or scary dreams can be emotional healing reactions during a sauna program. Many other natural therapies may help emotional healing.

Medications

If you take medical drugs, you may wish to ask your doctor if sauna therapy is all right. My experience is that saunas are safe with most drugs. Continue prescribed medication while doing sauna therapy, or discuss medication with the prescribing physician. Stopping insulin, heart medication, anti-seizure drugs, antibiotics or anti-depressant medications can have lethal consequences. Sauna therapy may reduce elevated blood pressure, and the need for other medication as well. However, it is best to consult your physician.

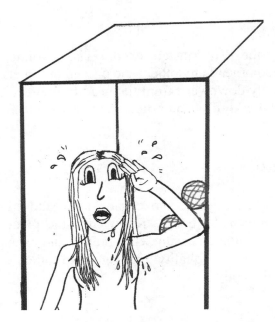

"It is so hot in here...it feels like I'm in a sauna."

8
Effects On Health Conditions

"I was diagnosed positive for HIV in 1987. As of January 2006, I have used an infrared lamp sauna for almost four years. My new blood work and physical examination are the best on record I have ever had since 1987! My T-cell count is 502 and normal on everything else. My cholesterol level is 142. That is with eating a lot of bacon and eggs, too. My HIV virus level is undetectable, even with the best instruments. - Mr. J. H., Palm Springs, CA

Sauna therapy can benefit hundreds of health conditions. The important areas of infections, general detoxification and cancer are covered in separate chapters.

This chapter discusses other health conditions for which there are some medical studies showing the effectiveness of sauna therapy. I hope this section will be expanded in the future as sauna therapy gains acceptance and receives more scientific scrutiny.

Cardiovascular System

Sauna therapy offers definite benefits for many cardiovascular conditions.

High Blood Pressure. Causes for elevated blood pressure include inflamed arteries, hidden infections, hardened arteries, constricted arteries and congestion of the kidneys. Sauna therapy can benefit all of these causes of high blood pressure.

Repeatedly shunting blood to the body surface with sauna therapy improves the flexibility of blood vessels, especially peripheral arteries. Deep tissue heating with infrared and eliminating toxic metals facilitates artery repair.

Sauna therapy is highly parasympathetic. This means that it helps relax the arterial muscles that are under autonomic nervous system control. Research indicates that sauna therapy can lead to decreased cardiac ejection resistance and decreased total peripheral resistance. This means that the arteries open up and blood flows through them more easily and with less pressure.

Heating the body several degrees, reducing sympathetic nervous system activity and many other mechanisms discussed in Chapter 9 help the body to alleviate infections that can contribute to inflammation of the arteries.

Enhancing elimination through the skin reduces the burden of detoxification of the kidneys. 'Essential' hypertension is often due in some measure to renal weakness and/or toxicity. The elimination of heavy metals such as mercury, lead and cadmium also assist kidney function. Heavy metal detoxification using sauna therapy often offers benefits superior to intravenous or oral chelation, though more time may be required using saunas.

Congestive Heart Failure. Recent research by T. Kihara and C. Tei show that spending time in a sauna can reduce symptoms associated with congestive heart failure. Spending 15 minutes a day, 5 days a week for two weeks reduced premature heartbeats, episodes of arrhythmia and levels of hormones linked to heart damage. These studies were conducted using infrared lamp saunas. Heat shock proteins produced as a result of sauna therapy may play an important role in improving congestive heart failure as well as recovery from heart attacks and other cardiovascular trauma. Cardiomyopathy has also responded well in one of my patients.

Atherosclerosis And Arteriosclerosis. Elimination of toxic metals such as iron, manganese, cadmium and other metals in the arteries, as occurs with chelation therapy as well, helps reduce inflammation and brittleness of the arteries. These are major causes of plaque formation. Sauna therapy can assist with this process, helping to improve flexibility of the arteries and discouraging plaque formation.

Cardiovascular Rehabilitation. Heating the body and repeatedly shunting the blood to the surface enhances oxygenation and encourages the formation of new blood vessels, assisting cardiovascular rehabilitation. Sauna therapy may also assist to restore flexibility to the arteries. Removing toxic metals and hidden infections can also greatly enhance cardiac function.

Multiple Chemical Sensitivity or MCS

Drs. Zane Gard, William Rea, David Root and many others have used the Hubbard method of detoxification using traditional saunas for several decades in some cases, with good results on patients with MCS.

The warmth of the sauna helps normalize body temperature and restore normal enzyme activity. Ridding the body of toxic metals, toxic chemicals and chronic infections is often a key to healing MCS. Improving circulation and oxygenation of the tissues are helpful to dislodge toxins as well as to facilitate their conversion to less toxic substances.

The relaxation afforded by saunas, particularly the low-temperature infrared type of saunas, may also be of therapeutic value. The nutrient value of infrared is also helpful for these patients. Highly allergic individuals may be unable to take nutritional supplements, but can usually tolerate and often love sauna baths. Shorter sessions may be needed at first.

Coil electric heaters and unshielded far infrared saunas may produce electromagnetic fields that are harmful for some very sensitive individuals. Infrared lamp saunas or gas-fired hot air saunas do not emit harmful electromagnetic fields.

Drug Detoxification

L. Ron Hubbard began using saunas for drug detoxification over 50 years ago. Detoxification clinics that use his system such as Narconon and others have treated over 500,000 people. Patients spend up to five hours per day in traditional hot air saunas under close supervision for two to three weeks or more.

Their program includes aerobic exercise for 20-30 minutes before a sauna session, use of high-dose niacin, electrolyte replacement, a wholesome diet and supplementary vitamins and minerals. Studies show good to excellent results with low recidivism rates.

The use of a near infrared lamp sauna with a nutritional balancing program may offer even more thorough tissue cleansing. I do not recommend niacin or exercise with sauna use.

Pesticide, Chemical And Toxic Metal Exposure

Medical studies indicate that saunas are of great benefit for those suffering from pesticide or other toxic chemical or heavy metal exposure. Many chemicals, as well as toxic metals, can be excreted through the skin. Enhancing circulation and oxygenation also helps release pesticides and other toxins from areas with poor circulation and can enhance the metabolic breakdown of toxic chemicals.

Enhancing skin elimination, normalizing enzyme activity, inhibiting the sympathetic nervous system and many other sauna therapy benefits all contribute to making it an excellent ways to rid our bodies of many toxic chemicals and heavy metals. Repeated sauna sessions for weeks or months are usually needed to fully activate the skin and allow the elimination of toxins that are lodged deeply within organs and other tissues.

Nervous System Disorders

Neurological conditions that may benefit from sauna therapy include *neuritis, neuralgia, facial paralysis, nerve root irritation* and many others. The heat of the sauna can penetrate into the brain and the rest of the nervous system, providing a means to help remove toxins and activate enzymes in this otherwise hard-to-reach but critical area of the body. Other sections of this book discuss in detail its powerful effects on the autonomic nervous system as well.

Psychological and emotional health conditions may also improve as brain chemistry normalizes. These may include *depression, anxiety, phobias* and *bipolar disorder*. ADHD, autism and others need to be the subject of greater research in the future.

Saunas are also excellent for general emotional well-being. Dr. P. Sorri, in his article entitled "The Sauna and Bathing Habits: A Psychoanalytic Point of View", wrote:

"The harsh world feels miles away and the bather lives in the here and now in the sauna...Many serious private and political problems have been constructively solved in the sauna. Rationality and commonplace thinking are abandoned and replaced by a positive disposition and an inclination to understand other people's point of view, thus promoting creativity and a capacity to find new solutions."

Books about saunas repeatedly mention that in many cultures the sauna or bath area is thought of as similar to an alter or holy place where one comes to meditate, pray and otherwise become peaceful and calm. My patients have commented similarly, one calling the sauna her "prayer box", where she retreats from distractions and is able to be centered and at peace.

Musculo-skeletal Conditions

Research from many nations indicates saunas are excellent for *muscle spasms, lumbar strain, sprains, tendonitis, bursitis*, many types of *pain, rheumatoid and osteoarthritis, whiplash, sciatica, soft tissue injuries* and *connective tissue disorders*.

Areas with poor circulation benefit greatly from tissue heating and improved blood flow. Saunas also act somewhat like a massage, forcibly shunting blood into and around muscles, ligaments and other soft tissues.

According to the text, *Therapeutic Heat and Cold*, heating enhances the flexibility of tendons and ligaments in ways that do not occur at normal body temperature. This may be helpful for a wide range of soft tissue injuries and conditions. Patients may find infrared saunas more beneficial due to their deep tissue penetration and greater comfort due to their lower operating temperatures.

Skin Conditions

All saunas help to open the pores, eliminate skin infections and toxins lodged in the skin, and restore elimination through the skin.

Near infrared, in particular, is excellent for *acne, eczema, psoriasis, burns, keloids and other scars, poor skin tone, diabetic skin ulcers, lacerations, dandruff, neurodermatitis, leg ulcers, wound healing, tattoo removal, postoperative edema* and *sun damage*. Other skin conditions often benefit as well from the enhanced circulation and the removal of toxic chemicals that build up in the skin.

Wound healing has been studied in greater depth by NASA and the military. A NASA report on light-emitting diodes (www.nasa.gov/vision/earth/technologies/led_treatment) states:

"Biologists have found that cells exposed to near-infrared light – that is, energy just outside the visible range – from leds (light-emitting diodes) grow 150-200% faster than those cells not stimulated by such light. This form of light increases energy inside cells which results in speeding up the healing process...

Infrared, especially near infrared in the 600-1000 nm range, promotes fibroblast proliferation, enhances chondroplasia, upregulates the synthesis of type I and type II procollagen mRNA, quickens bone repair and remodeling, fosters revascularization of wounds and overall accelerates tissue repair in experimental and clinical models". (Therapeutic Light, *Rehab. Management*, Jan/Feb 2004)

Ear, Nose and Throat Conditions

Japanese research with infrared indicates benefits for *chronic middle ear infections, sore throats, ringing in the ears and nose bleeds. Sinus conditions* are extremely common and often chronic due to poor circulation in this area, impairing the ability of medications to reach the area.

Sauna therapy and the use of a single isolated infrared lamp on the area we find most helpful for healing *acute* and *chronic sinus conditions*. However, very chronic sinus, ear and other infections may require several weeks, months or even more than a year of repeated sauna

72

use for complete healing to occur. A healthful lifestyle and plenty of rest are also important along with sauna therapy.

Eye Conditions

Infrared in particular may be very beneficial for the eyes. While more research is needed in this areas, Nature Science Update, March 2003 reported that exposure to near infrared light was beneficial for rats with *methanol-induced blindness*, a common cause of accidental blindness (*Proc Natl Acad Sci.*, 2003, doi:10.1073/pnas.0534736100, March 7).

Most people can and should keep their eyes open in an infrared lamp sauna, although we do not recommend staring directly at the lamps.

Digestive Disorders

Sauna therapy inhibits the sympathetic nervous system, which tends to enhance the activity of the digestive system. Saunas can therefore add energy to the "digestive fire" in the belly and they promote greater circulation in the abdominal area.

Studies have reported improvement in many digestive conditions including cases of *gastroenteritis, diarrhea, constipation, cholecystitis, candida albicans and other parasitic infections, dysbiosis, diverticulosis, diverticulitis, ulcers, colitis, hemorrhoids, pancreatitis* and *intestinal cancers*. Not all these of these improvements have been proven as yet in double-blind medical studies, however, in part because of the difficulty of doing these studies with sauna therapy. How, after all, can research subjects not know when they are undergoing sauna therapy? This is one of the problems of requiring double-blind studies before medical science will accept the value of a procedure such as sauna therapy

Reproductive Conditions

While I do not recommend saunas longer than 10 minutes during pregnancy until proven safe by modern research methods, saunas may be helpful for a variety of female organ conditions for the same reasons they help digestive disorders. That is, the sauna's heat moves the body into a more parasympathetic state, greatly assists circulation to the area and increases the yang or fire energy in the lower abdomen.

More research is needed. However, conditions that may benefit from sauna therapy include *pelvic inflammatory disease, other pelvic infections including sexually transmitted diseases, fibroid tumors, ovarian and uterine cysts and tumors, menstrual pain* and *menopausal symptoms*.

Other

Saunas may also benefit *varicose veins, multiple sclerosis, lupus, chronic fatigue, adhesions, pneumonia* and *many acute and chronic infections*.

Much more research is needed as physicians who use sauna therapy find that gentle heating of the body, especially with infrared energy, is an excellent prescription for many health conditions.

One never knows to what extent the presence of chronic infections or excessive amounts of toxic metals and toxic chemicals contribute to ill health. Clearing these from the body and enhancing skin elimination help restore basic metabolic and biochemical integrity that will benefit an enormous number of health conditions.

9
Saunas And Infectious Disease

I have had Lyme disease for the past 25 years. We installed an infrared lamp sauna in a wardrobe according to Dr. Wilson's instructions six weeks ago. My blood pressure has gone from a pathetic 80/50 up to nearly normal 110/70! My doctor is amazed. I have informed many others who are battling with "incurable" neurally-mediated hypotension.

I have also managed to do five weeks of voluntary work, which involves standing on my feet for several hours. I use a walking frame intermittently, but previously I would have to lie down frequently and could only cope for a couple of hours. God bless you. - Mrs. R.V., Australia

A number of studies have been published demonstrating the effectiveness of saunas for alleviating infections. Patients report the infrared lamp sauna has cleared chronic infected teeth as well as infections of the sinuses, bronchial tubes, eyes, ears, throat, lungs, intestines, bladder and many others.

Two basic approaches for preventing and overcoming infections are 1) improving the resistance of the host and 2) disabling or killing pathogenic microorganisms. Sauna therapy combines a number of mechanisms to accomplish both these objectives.

Heating The Body

Heating, as occurs in fever, is a natural mechanism to disable microorganisms. Many bacteria, fungi, parasites (including the spirochetes of Lyme disease) and cells infected with viruses, are weaker than normal cells and more susceptible to damage by heat. The sauna can raise body temperature several degrees, facilitating control and elimination of these microorganisms. Mark Konlee, author of the *Immune Restoration Handbook*, wrote:

"Temperatures even 1° below 98.6° F. indicate impaired white blood cell response to infections...No treatment for any chronic infection will ever be completely satisfactory until body temperature returns to normal".

Most adults have a low body temperature, usually due to impaired adrenal and thyroid glandular activity. This prevents them from making use of the germ-killing effects of fever. Saunas are particularly helpful for these individuals. The needed heat is provided without any effort required on the part of the body. With continued therapy, glandular activity often improves, alleviating the problem of low body temperature.

Improving Circulation

Impaired circulation is a factor in many infections, especially in tissues with poor circulation. Saunas quickly, safely and powerfully improve circulation as blood is forced to the surface in the body's attempt to get rid of extra heat. Areas with poor circulation include the joints, sinuses, bones and extremities. These are frequently sites of chronic infections, which may be helped by sauna therapy. However, improved circulation helps with most any infection.

Improved Oxygenation

Many bacteria, fungi and other pathogens are anaerobic organisms. This means they do not thrive in an oxygen-rich environment. Impaired oxygenation is common today due to poor circulation, muscle tension, toxic metals, toxic chemicals and shallow respiration.

Improved oxygenation due to sauna therapy weakens many pathogens. At the same time, it promotes oxygen-dependent cellular processes needed to fight infections.

Sweating

For infections of the skin such as acne, impetigo, eczema and others, sweating cleanses the skin from the inside. This facilitates the removal of bacteria, chemicals and cellular debris from deep within the skin that contribute to many skin infections. An exception may be rosacea. A patient reported that infrared sauna use aggravated his case of rosacea.

Effects of Infrared Radiation

Infrared radiation is highly compatible with human physiology. It acts as a nutrient, enhancing cellular energy production and cell respiration. These benefits assist the body to both resist and heal many types of infections.

Deep Heat Penetration

Infrared saunas, especially infrared lamp saunas, directly heat the tissues from the inside. This is an excellent extra benefit of infrared for reaching internal infections in areas with poor circulation such as the sinuses, bladder, ears, nasal passages, throat and many other sites. Deep

76

tissue heating also assists to raise the body temperature sufficiently to disable microorganisms and perhaps to produce heat shock proteins.

Sympathetic Nervous System Inhibition

Fatigue, stress, unhealthful lifestyles, toxic conditions and nutritional depletion can all stimulate the sympathetic branch of the autonomic nervous system. This in turn stimulates cortisol production that suppresses immune system activity.

"Cortisol decreases the number of eosinophils and lymphocytes (and) decreases the output of both lymphocytes and antibodies from the lymphoid tissue. As a result, the level of immunity for almost all foreign invaders of the body is decreased. This can occasionally lead to fulminating infection and death from diseases that otherwise would not be lethal." (Guyton, p. 951).

Sauna therapy inhibits sympathetic nervous system activity. This enhances the activity of the immune system.

Production of Heat Shock Proteins

Heat shock proteins have been shown to be powerful immune system stimulators. They can restore normal cellular immune system activity and help the body recognize and destroy infectious agents.

Heating the body several degrees, as can occur with sauna therapy, may be one of the best ways to safely produce heat shock proteins.

Enhancing Digestion

Many nutrients are needed for the immune system. Excessive stress and sympathetic nervous stimulation diminish digestive activity. Saunas enhance the digestion and absorption of many nutrients essential for immune system activation.

Light and Color Therapy

The use of visible light frequencies for healing is a separate topic that could occupy an entire volume. Light frequencies produced by the infrared lamp sauna and which can be added to any sauna will enhance the germ-killing and tissue-repairing effects of the sauna. The extensive benefits of phototherapy for infections are presented in *Into the Light* and texts by Dinshaw Ghadiali and Darius Dinshaw such as *Let There Be Light*.

Color therapy in the infrared lamp sauna with the red, orange and yellow spectrum is stimulating. However, it supports the activity of the liver, kidneys, intestines, pancreas and other parasympathetic organs, which in turn help activate aspects of the immune system.

No Side Effects or Tolerance

Antibiotics, antiviral agents and other drugs may cause nutrient depletion and liver and kidney toxicity, actually weakening one's immune system. Also, bacteria and other microorganisms eventually develop tolerance to their use. Vaccines that worked against older strains of smallpox, anthrax and other diseases may not have any effect on newer genetically altered strains of disease.

Sauna therapy is very safe, with literally thousands of years of testing. Its only 'side effect' is improved overall health. It does not cause the development of resistant organisms and, for this reason, will likely be effective for new strains of pathogenic organisms. This makes it suitable for a wide range of infections and safe for most everyone when used wisely.

Combining With Other Therapies

If antibiotics or other medications are needed, sauna therapy can be used at the same time without fear. This cannot be said of some drug combinations and certain other therapies, which can result in extreme toxicity.

Inexpensive and Available to All

Drug therapy can run several hundred dollars or more. A lamp sauna that can be used by an entire family, or even an entire neighborhood, can be built for under $300.00 and operated for pennies a day.

Therapy can also be done safely at home, even when ill. These cost factors make it widely accessible to people everywhere, including those without access to modern medicines or the funds to pay for them.

Sauna Use In Acute Infections

These include colds, flu, sore throats, sinus infections, dysentery and others. Use the sauna *aggressively*. The most common error is not using it enough or waiting too long before starting therapy. Waiting can cause complications to develop.

With acute infections, use the sauna more often for shorter periods of time. Use the sauna for about 10 minutes, about four to nine times a day *at the first sign of infection*. Often one can stop an infection before it develops further. If, however, an infection is not responding to one's efforts after 4-5 days, be sure to consult a competent professional. The following are also most helpful:

1. Absolute bed rest. Conserve energy for healing. Stay home from work. Children should be kept home from school and in bed or at least lying down when ill. Continuing to work or sending sick children to school is asking for complications.

2. Eat lightly. Soups, liquids or small quantities of food should be all that is taken. Most people have little appetite when ill. A fast with just water or water with lemon for up to three days may be helpful, especially if fever is present.

3. Stop taking a full complement of nutritional supplements. One may continue digestive aids, fiber, and calcium and magnesium. Herbs, especially *echinacea, astralagus, medicinal mushrooms, bee propolis* and *olive leaf extract* may be helpful. *Vitamin A* up to 150,000 iu daily for a week is often helpful. *Zinc* and *vitamin C* may also be helpful. *High-quality colloidal silver, tea tree oil* and other essential oils may also be excellent.

4. Lower fever only if it is above 103° F with a sponge bath, and preferably NOT with Tylenol or aspirin. A sponge bath allows the body to keep producing heat, which can speed recovery. Tylenol is quite toxic and its overuse is a major cause of liver failure today.

5. Other natural therapies include enemas, colonic irrigation, deep breathing, foot massage, energy balancing, visualization and homeopathic remedies.

Saunas Use For Chronic Infections

Most people have at least a dozen chronic infections. I did not believe this until I began experimenting with lamp sauna therapy. Common sites are the sinuses, ears, eyes, skin, bladder, kidneys, lungs, bronchial tubes, teeth, bone, gums, intestines, tendons and ligaments. Many conditions such as asthma, vertigo, post-nasal drip, vague aches and pains, vaginal discharges, eczema, artery disease, ulcers and fatigue may be due to chronic, low-grade infections.

Impaired energy, poor circulation, a low body temperature and the presence of antibiotic residues combine to set the stage for chronic infections. Toxicity with copper, mercury, cadmium, arsenic, lead, iron and manganese also weaken the body. Autonomic imbalance and nutritional deficiencies may prevent healing of chronic infections.

Eliminating chronic infections is a major benefit of prolonged sauna therapy. A year or more of daily sauna sessions is often required to uncover and promote their healing.

All types of saunas are helpful to eliminate chronic infections. I find the most powerful is an infrared lamp sauna. This type heats tissues more deeply, provides a wide spectrum of healing frequencies and one can focus the rays on a part of the body that needs attention. An infrared lamp sauna may be as much as ten times as powerful for chronic infections as a hot air sauna or a far infrared ceramic element sauna. My personal experience with chronic infections is detailed in Chapter 14.

Epidemics And Pandemics

Many people are concerned about the avian flu, the West Nile virus, Hanta virus and other potentially lethal infections for which few means exist to combat them. Sauna therapy offers an inexpensive and safe approach that may prove vital if an epidemic of great proportions should ever occur.

Saunas Versus Vaccination. Vaccination is often recommended for these and other infectious diseases, if a vaccine is even available. Problems with vaccines that are often overlooked include: 1) they may not work, especially if disease strains are genetically altered, 2) they may have serious side effects, 3) the need for them is often exaggerated. Vaccines are *not* the cause of the eradication of smallpox, tuberculosis, polio and other diseases. This is well documented (see the Millbank Memorial Fund Quarterly, Summer 1977, pp. 405-428).

As an aside, I feel that the risk of a pandemic flu or other outbreak is somewhat overstated. Dr. Tom Mack, a researcher at the University of Southern California, recently spoke at a Centers for Disease Control *Public Forum on Smallpox*. His credentials include spending more time working with smallpox outbreaks than anyone else in Pakistan and other nations. He said,

"If there were a terrorist attack, I would expect a small number of cases. I think that airborne spread would be relatively inefficient and I don't think very many cases would occur... Fatality is usually less than advertised ...probably around 10-15 percent... If people are worried about endemic smallpox, it disappeared from this country not because of our mass herd immunity. It disappeared because of our economic development. That's why it disappeared from Europe and many other countries...and it will not be sustained here, even if there were several importations."

Saunas are excellent to alleviate infectious diseases due to viruses as well as bacteria, fungi and other microorganisms. I hope this text encourages the reader to consider sauna therapy before rushing to potentially lethal and ineffective vaccine programs to protect oneself and others from infectious diseases.

10
Saunas and Cancer

"I am a consultant who works with metabolic cancer therapy. I have found infrared lamp sauna therapy to be extremely beneficial for my patients. It has allowed us to save many more lives and greatly reduce the time needed for detoxification. I recommend the infrared lamp sauna for all patients undergoing metabolic cancer therapy. I used other types of saunas but did not achieve the same results." - R.T., Denver, CO

Sauna therapy can be an excellent addition to any biological or metabolic cancer therapy program. Saunas may also help patients undergoing conventional chemotherapy. The infrared lamp sauna appears most helpful. However, I am not aware of any formal studies on the subject. Infrared lamp sauna benefits for cancer include:

- Assisting the removal of chemical toxins and heavy metals.
- Increasing oxygenation and circulation.
- Enhancing the immune system.
- Inhibiting the sympathetic nervous system.
- Reducing the radiation burden in the body (Yamazaki, 1987).
- Uncovering and healing chronic infections. Endo- and exotoxins from chronic infections in the teeth and elsewhere often contribute to the development of cancer.

What is Cancer?

In 1902, Dr. John Beard published a paper in *The Lancet* on the trophoblastic theory of cancer (Beard, J., 1902). It is quite simple and has never been disproven. In fact, it recently received strong confirmation by scientists at the University of Michigan (Townsend Letter, #240, 2003). Dr. Beard showed that a normal tissue of the body, the trophoblast, exhibits characteristics identical to cancer. It is invasive, metastatic, forms new blood vessels (angiogenesis) and has the same specific markers and chemical composition as cancer cells.

The trophoblast is a totipotent or stem cell that grows around the developing fetus during the first eight to twelve weeks of pregnancy. The word trophoblast means 'nourishing the baby'.

It burrows into the lining of the mother's uterus and supplies the fetus with blood until the placenta forms. It is essential for life.

The trophoblast normally disappears between 8 and 12 weeks of pregnancy. If it overgrows, the result is a very virulent form of cancer, choriocarcinoma. It usually kills both mother and fetus within a few weeks.

One may say, if the trophoblast only develops during pregnancy, how can it explain all other cancers? Dr. Beard found that the stem cells that form the trophoblast are present all over the body in small numbers. Given the right stimulus, they begin to grow. A key to understanding cancer is to understand what makes these cells grow.

Estrogen, A Primary Carcinogen

The primary stimulus for the growth of the trophoblast is high estrogen, as occurs during pregnancy. Estrogen is associated with cell proliferation. Modern medicine acknowledges that estrogen is a carcinogen, for which reason estrogen inhibitors are among the drugs used for cancer.

One may ask, why does so much cancer occur in men, or in post-menopausal women who do not produce as much estrogen? The answer is that everyone's adrenal glands and perhaps other sites produce estrogens, in both sexes and at all ages.

Normal estrogen production by the adrenal glands or ovaries is not a problem. The liver converts the potent estrogens such as estrone to a harmless form. However, when the liver is toxic or otherwise compromised, it cannot detoxify estrogen properly. Estrone increases and the stage is set for cancer. Guyton explains the fate of the estrogens as follows:

> "The liver conjugates the estrogens ... and about one-fifth of these conjugated products are excreted in the bile while most of the remainder are excreted in the urine. Also, the liver converts the potent estrogens, estradiol and estrone, into an almost impotent estrogen, estriol. Therefore, the liver plays an important role in removing those estrogens from the blood. *Indeed, diminished liver function actually increases activity of estrogens in the body, sometimes causing hyperestrinism.*" (Guyton, p.1010) (italics are mine)

Liver toxicity today is the rule rather then the exception. Causes for liver toxicity include:

- **Toxins in the food supply.** These include toxic metals, pesticide residues, preservatives and thousands of other additives used in prepared foods. Some pesticides and other chemicals mimic the effects of estrogen by occupying estrogen binding sites. This may cause more estrogens to circulate freely in the body. An interesting recent study found that cadmium mimics the effects of estrogen (*Nature*, August 2003).

- **Thousands of organic chemicals and toxic metals in the environment.** Besides food, sources of toxins include contaminated air, dental materials, especially silver amalgam fillings, and skin contact with toxins in solvents, detergents, skin care products, chlorinated and fluoridated water and other household and industrial chemicals. Building materials, carpets, plastics and office machinery may also outgas toxic chemicals.

82

- **Radiation exposure damages the liver.** Everyone is exposed to some ionizing radiation from bomb fallout, nuclear plant accidents, medical x-rays and other uses of radiation.

- **Prescription, over-the-counter and other remedies.** Almost all pharmaceuticals are synthetic chemicals that must be detoxified and excreted, primarily by the liver. Drug residues are present even in tap water supplies. Vaccines may be preserved with toxic metals. Many herbs are toxic as well, though much less than most drugs. Vitamin products that contain sea minerals and land-based mineral deposits often contain toxic metals. A portion of any ingested drug or chemical remains in the body, often for years. These will build up and can be an important source of liver toxicity.

- **Adrenal exhaustion.** This is an indirect cause. Adrenal weakness contributes to a slow oxidation rate and sluggish liver activity. Also, the body compensates for adrenal depletion by accumulating toxic levels of copper, iron, chromium, selenium, manganese, aluminum, cadmium, iron, lead and other metals that are toxic to the liver.

- **Nutrient deficiencies.** Most people have nutrient deficiencies. These impair the liver's normal detoxification pathways. Nutrient deficiencies are the result of poor quality diets, poor eating habits and impaired digestion. Also, stress increases the need for nutrients.

- **Impaired digestion.** Poor digestion causes the production of toxic substances in the intestines due to fermentation and putrefaction of food. A vicious cycle occurs in which the toxic liver does not produce enough bile and digestive enzymes. Food is then poorly digested, which generates toxins that in turn worsen the condition of the liver. This further impairs enzyme production, which results in more toxins in the intestines.

- **Improper bowel flora such as candida albicans and other pathogenic organisms.** These can produce deadly toxins in the intestines. Candida albicans, for example, produces alcohol and acetaldehyde.

- **Chronic infections anywhere in the body.** Bacterial and other infections generate endotoxins and exotoxins. Chronic infections are much more common than imagined. I estimate most people have a dozen low-grade chronic infections. Common sites are the teeth, eyes, ears, throat, bladder, bronchials, intestines and skin.

- **Stress from any cause activates the sympathetic nervous system, which in turn reduces liver activity.** Stress also impairs digestion, which leads to more toxin generation in the intestines.

- **Autonomic imbalance, in particular excessive sympathetic nervous system activity.** The sympathetic nervous system inhibits the activity of the liver. This is explained below in more detail.

- **Fatigue.** Fatigue can be an important factor in liver toxicity.

Sauna therapy can be most helpful for many of these imbalances. It helps with detoxification, chronic infections, inhibiting the sympathetic nervous system, decongesting the internal organs and improving circulation. Sauna therapy thus can assist with several mechanisms that inhibit abnormal trophoblast activity.

Reduced Pancreatic Enzyme Secretion

At about 12 weeks of pregnancy, the trophoblast usually stops growing and the placenta takes over the function of nourishing the fetus. Dr. Beard found that enzymes produced by the fetal and maternal pancreas stop the growth of the trophoblast.

This is the basis for the use of pancreatic enzymes in the treatment of cancer advocated by Dr. William Kelley, DDS and others (Kelley, W.D., 1997). Large quantities of pancreatic enzymes are given by mouth, which inhibit the growth of malignant cells.

The pancreas plays another role. Pancreatic enzymes are needed for proper digestion. A weakened, toxic or depleted pancreas contributes to a toxic liver by failing to provide adequate enzymes for complete food digestion. Many people do not produce enough pancreatic enzymes or they overeat, exceeding their digestive capacity. These pancreatic enzymes are not the same as "food enzymes" found in raw food. Ideally, excess pancreatic enzymes are secreted so that any cancer that begins to develop will be destroyed.

Causes for deficient pancreatic activity are similar to the causes of liver toxicity. They include stress, poor-quality diets, poor eating habits, infections and toxic exposures. For this reason, sauna therapy can be most helpful to restore pancreatic activity.

The Role Of The Autonomic Nervous System

An important cause of impaired pancreas and liver activity is excessive activity of the sympathetic nervous system. This branch of the autonomic nervous system is sometimes referred to as the fight-or-flight response system. It prepares the body for a stress response and inhibits the activity of the liver, kidneys, pancreas, intestines and stomach. These are the organs of detoxification and the organs needed to produce digestive enzymes and cancer-fighting proteolytic enzymes (enzymes that digest foreign proteins).

Excessive activity of the sympathetic nervous system is extremely common today. Causes include stress, hurried or busy lifestyles, toxic metals, nutrient deficiencies, some toxic chemicals and negative attitudes such as fear, worry, anger, resentment and guilt. These factors keep the body in a fight-or-flight or sympathetic state.

Many cancer patients have a sympathetic dominant personality. This means they have difficulty relaxing and are often hard on themselves and others. They are often fearful, angry, guilty, perfectionistic, resentful or use other mechanisms that cause the body to remain in a sympathetic state much of the time. People who exercise too much, worry a lot, work too hard or are obsessive often overwork the sympathetic nervous system.

Therapies that inhibit the sympathetic nervous system are marvelous for cancer patients. These include saunas, coffee enemas, colon therapy, pancreatic enzyme therapy and minerals including calcium, magnesium and zinc. Lots of rest, relaxation techniques, meditation, bodywork, biofeedback and other methods are also helpful.

84

Sauna Mechanisms For Cancer

The key to the use of sauna therapy for cancer is it combines some dozen or so therapeutic mechanisms that act together in concert to inhibit tumor growth and strengthen the body. These include:

1. Heating The Body. Hyperthermia is a known method of killing cancer cells. Cancer cells are weaker than normal cells and more susceptible to damage from heat.

Saunas are not the same as hypothermia that heats the body up to 104-105° F. However, sauna therapy, if repeated several times daily, is a safe, gentle and more easily controlled method of heating the tissues that may have a hyperthermic effect. Infrared saunas are most likely better for this purpose as they heat the tissues directly. Far infrared saunas heat to about an inch and a half inside the body. Infrared lamp saunas with three 250-watt lamps heat up to about three inches inside the body.

2. Inhibiting The Sympathetic Nervous System. The sympathetic branch of the autonomic nervous system activates the brain, muscles, thyroid and adrenal glands to respond to stress. It also tends to inhibit the activity of the eliminative organs and the immune system.

Excessive activity of the sympathetic nervous system may contribute to many cases of cancer. Therapies that inhibit the sympathetic system are helpful and at times critical for cancer recovery. Sauna therapy is helpful for this purpose.

At least three sauna mechanisms inhibit the sympathetic nervous system:

- Heating the body reduces normal heat production, a sympathetic activity. (Guyton, P. 892)
- Saunas draw blood from the center to the periphery of the body, a parasympathetic activity.
- Saunas also help eliminate from the body minerals and chemical compounds that can keep the body in a sympathetic state. These include mercury, aluminum, cadmium, lead and excessive or toxic forms of iron, copper, manganese and other minerals. They also include some pesticides and other toxic chemicals.

3. Improving Circulation. Cancer often grows in tissues with poor circulation and thus poor nutrition and oxygenation. In its effort to remove the heat of the sauna, the body powerfully shunts blood to the skin and increases the heart rate. This combination has a powerful stimulating effect on circulation. This helps bring needed nutrients, hormones, oxygen and other substances to all body tissues and to drain off cellular waste products.

4. Decongesting The Internal Organs. Congestion of the liver, kidneys and other internal organs inhibits the detoxification of estrogen and the elimination of toxic chemicals and heavy metals. By increasing the blood circulation and causing blood to move toward the body surface, sauna therapy can help decongest the internal organs.

5. Possibly Producing Heat Shock Proteins. Heat shock proteins are a discovery of the past 20-30 years (Kukreja, 2000, Verlag, 1991). These interesting substances are produced naturally by the body when it is subjected to certain stressors, among them heat. Heat shock proteins can renature normal cellular proteins, which means to repair and rebuild damaged cell structures. They are being studied in cancer research laboratories as they have been found to be potent immune system boosters. Infrared sauna therapy may be a simple and safe way to induce natural production of heat shock proteins.

"When HSPs encounter tumor fragments, they pack them up for processing by the immune system's defensive macrophage cells, setting in motion a chain of events that results in the recognition of the tumor. The body's cytotoxic T-lymphocytes (also known as killer T-cells) then attack the cancer cells that produced the material sponged up by the HSPs. The tumor is thus killed even without the ability to recognize individual epitopes (surface characteristics of cancer cells that allow the immune system to identify it as dangerous). This natural process has been used successfully in vaccinations of mice and rats with experimental tumors." (see *Heat Shock Proteins: New Avenues to Cancer Vaccines*)

6. Infrared Benefits. Infrared helps decouple toxins from water molecules, acts as a nutrient and enhances cell regeneration. These benefits are likely to occur most with the use of an infrared lamp sauna, which offers a wide spectrum of near, medium and a little far infrared energy. According to Japanese research, infrared may also enhance oxygen production within the cells (*Jap J Inflammation*, November 1996, 16(6):9).

Infrared resonates at the frequency of water and increases the normal activity of water molecules in the cells. It also reduces the specific gravity of water so that it penetrates cells better, carrying more nutrients to the cells and helping remove toxins from the cells.

7. Enhancing Oxygenation. Oxygen therapies may be helpful for cancer as cancer thrives in an anaerobic environment. Saunas enhance oxygenation several ways. They increase blood flow through the lungs and the skin, assisting the blood to pick up more oxygen. They also increase circulation to all body tissues, distributing more oxygen to all the tissues. Saunas may also help remove toxic metals and chemicals that can cause an *anemia of chronic disease* that can reduce the oxygen-carrying capacity of the blood. Among these toxins are lead, copper, mercury, arsenic and cyanide.

8. Balancing The pH. Saunas may help balance both an excessively acid and an excessively alkaline body chemistry. This occurs due to improved circulation and oxygenation, enhanced cellular nutrition and correcting the metabolic rate.

9. Genetic Effects. Genetics researchers often forget to mention that nutrients turn on genes, while nutrient deficiencies and toxins can alter or block genetic expression. Infrared lamp sauna therapy may help improve cellular DNA by several mechanisms:

- It can help remove radioactive particles bound to metals or other toxic chemicals.
- The sauna's heat may disable or even kill heat-sensitive cells mutated by radiation that otherwise would reproduce.

10. Color Therapy. Color therapy is greatly underrated. Red, yellow and orange light, produced by an infrared lamp sauna, nourish the lower chakras and the organs of elimination including the liver, kidneys and large intestine (Dinshaw, 2005). Color therapy can be added to any sauna and is an excellent adjunct to sauna therapy.

One may also add other colored lights to any sauna. The science of color therapy is ancient and is an area for future research.

Saunas and the Mental State

Maintaining a positive mental attitude is very important for cancer patients. Many patients report that sauna therapy feels good, is relaxing and leaves them refreshed and happier. Some report that the quiet and privacy of the sauna is like a gift to oneself that they cherish. In the sauna, one can shut out the cares of the day.

A sauna session can also be used as a spiritual and meditative time that is set aside each day to reaffirm one's bond with the creator.

Tumor Necrosis, Pain Control and Ascites

In addition to metal and chemical toxicity, cancer patients must deal with toxicity due to the disintegration or necrosis of tumors that occurs with natural healing therapies.

Tumors may also swell as they disintegrate. This may help dilute toxins released from dying cells. This can put pressure on another organ or structure that may require extra attention. Extra coffee enemas are extremely helpful and at times life-saving if symptoms of detoxification become intense.

Patients report that sauna therapy has proven helpful for the pain of cancer. It may also assist in advanced cases with the management of ascites and other complications.

Other Therapy Considerations

Converting Saunas. While any sauna may help a cancer patient, the best sauna for cancer patients appears to be the infrared lamp sauna.

Plans for this type of sauna using hardware store parts are found in Appendix D. One can also buy an inexpensive tent type of lamp sauna that works excellently. If one has a different type of sauna, it can often convert easily to the infrared light type by adding infrared lamps. See Chapter 13 for details on converting a sauna to an infrared lamp sauna.

Preheating. To produce the maximum heat shock proteins for immune stimulation, I suggest preheating the sauna for 20 minutes so that it will be hotter during the session. Allow an infrared lamp sauna to reach 120° F. Hotter than this is not necessary or helpful. The only caution is that sauna therapy may have to be regulated according to the ability of the patient to tolerate it. If debilitated, begin with short sessions.

Sauna Cancer Protocol. It is important to be relaxed during sauna sessions to obtain the maximum benefit. For this reason, the best times for saunas are first thing in the morning and last thing at night. For cancer patients, a third and perhaps even a fourth session may be in late morning and/or afternoon. Each session may need to be shorter, such as 20-30 minutes, especially if one is debilitated. Do coffee enemas *after* sauna sessions.

Rest 15-20 minutes after a sauna session to achieve the maximum benefit. Drinking enough water and adding kelp granules or tablets to one's nutritional regimen is usually all that is required to replace electrolytes lost during sweating.

A simple way to determine the correct amount of water needed after a sauna session is to weigh oneself before and after a session. Then drink enough to replace the weight lost during the session. A quart of water weighs two pounds.

Showering after each sauna session is most helpful. Some people do not want to take the time to shower. However, one will reabsorb some toxins if they remain on the skin too long. Use a skin brush each time one showers and reduce soap and shampoo use as much as possible. If showering is difficult or inconvenient, wipe off the body well with a clean, moist towel.

Duration of Sauna Therapy. On average, at least three years of continuous sauna therapy are recommended for cancer cases. One will often feel better much sooner. However, since cancer is an end-stage illness, three years are best to prevent a recurrence. After this, assuming health has returned and tests are normal, I recommend maintenance sauna use with about three sessions per week.

Supervision. If one is debilitated, have an attendant or friend present while in the sauna, at least at the beginning of a sauna program until one is completely familiar with sauna use. Also, during treatment, one's energy will vary as toxins are released and body chemistry shifts. It is most helpful to have someone else present if feeling very debilitated.

Saunas During Healing Reactions. Those on natural cancer therapy programs will experience healing reactions or flare-ups. These are normal and often positive signs that healing at deep levels is proceeding. Often one is eliminating toxic metals or chemicals.

At these times, it is often helpful to reduce the duration of sauna sessions. More frequent, shorter sauna sessions are generally preferable during a healing reaction. In some cases, saunas may have to be suspended for a few days if healing reactions are intense. However, most people tolerate and benefit from short sessions, even 10 minutes or less, throughout healing reactions. More supervision is always helpful at these times.

Dental Amalgams and Root Canals. In an effort to detoxify the body quickly, many holistic physicians recommend removing dental amalgams when one has cancer. Dr. William Kelley and others have asserted very strongly that this is a bad idea. The extra toxins released during the procedure, even when the best protocol for removal is followed, often kill the patient. It is best to leave the mercury amalgams alone until the patient is better.

Root Canals. These are often a source of very toxic bacteria for cancer patients and the general population alike. Removing root canals does not appear to traumatize cancer patients. Removal can be very important for healing if the root canals are infected, as they often are.

11
Healing Reactions

"After using an infrared lamp sauna daily for about three months, I developed intense pain and swelling of my jaw next to two lower teeth. A dental x-ray confirmed two abscessed teeth and the dentist recommended antibiotics and immediate removal of the affected teeth. However, I was told this was likely a healing reaction and to continue with sauna therapy twice daily and use a single infrared lamp for five minutes at a time every hour during the day. In three days, the abscess burst open inside my mouth. The pain disappeared completely and the teeth have been fine for over two years." - Mr. E. F., Prescott, AZ

Healing reactions are temporary symptoms associated with eliminating toxic substances, healing chronic infections or due to other metabolic changes in the body. *They are an important feature of all deep healing methods.* They are usually mild, benign and short-lived, and one feels much better afterwards. Occasionally they are vigorous, unpleasant and even frightening. In fact, however, they are welcome signs of healing. If they did not occur with sauna therapy, we would know that this method does not produce healing at deep levels.

Healing reactions are not a new idea at all. Textbooks of medicine, chiropractic and other natural healing sciences refer to them as *flare-ups, retracing reactions, catharsis, purification reactions, the reversal process* or *exacerbations*. Max Gerson, MD, in *A Cancer Therapy - Results of 50 Cases*, devoted an entire chapter to them. He called them flare-ups. William Frederich Koch, MD mentions them often in his excellent book, *The Survival Factor in Neoplastic and Viral Diseases*. Bernard Jensen, DC, ND wrote about them in *The Doctor-Patient Handbook*.

Healing reactions are little understood in allopathic medical practice, so many people are unfamiliar with them. However, they are very important to understand if one is to undergo sauna therapy, and especially if guiding others through sauna therapy programs. One needs to understand why these reactions occur, how to distinguish them from a worsening of a disease condition and how to discuss them and handle them safely.

Why Healing Reactions Occur

As toxins are mobilized from storage sites throughout the body, they are transported by the blood to the liver primarily, and in some instances elsewhere. Once they reach the organs of elimination, which include the liver, colon, kidneys, skin and lungs primarily, they must be processed through these organs to be eliminated from the body. Symptoms can arise for many reasons:

- Toxic metals and chemicals circulating in the blood may cause headaches and many other symptoms until they are eliminated. The exact symptom varies depending on the nature of the toxin.
- The liver, kidneys, skin or lungs can become temporarily overloaded by the amount of toxins being processed, resulting in symptoms.
- Bile containing toxins dumped into the small intestine often causes temporary diarrhea or abdominal distress.
- Release of toxins can uncover old chronic infections, which may release endotoxins causing a flare-up of pain or other symptoms.
- Metabolic changes due to toxin release may cause a temporary reduction or increase in thyroid or adrenal hormone secretion. This, in turn, can cause temporary symptoms related to the blood sugar or energy level, or the ability to sleep, and may cause mental or emotional changes as well.
- Nutrient levels can shift quickly during healing reactions. Some are used as chelators and others, such as sulfur and zinc, are eliminated with toxic substances. Others act as buffers during toxin elimination. Others replace toxic metals, such as zinc replacing cadmium or copper in certain enzymes or magnesium replacing mercury. Other nutrients such as selenium are used to make more glutathione needed for detoxification. These shifts in critical nutrient levels may result in temporary symptoms until levels stabilize once again.
- Thousands of enzymes depend on vital minerals and are poisoned by toxic metals and chemical toxins. As the toxins are released, the activity of some enzymes, as well as the amounts of hormones, neurotransmitters and other cellular activators may shift. This can result in almost any symptom imaginable until homeostasis is restored. Rebalancing usually takes just minutes or hours, but can take longer in some instances.

Symptoms of Healing Reactions

Most healing reactions are mild and pass quickly. Symptoms may include diarrhea, constipation, aches, pains, muscle cramps, discharges, odors, rashes, headaches, irritability and fatigue. While these are the most common ones, almost any physical symptom may occur. Emotional reactions may include feelings of anxiety, depression, moodiness, crying, fear or anger.

Most symptoms are mild and transitory. Rest and reassurance are usually all that are required to pass through them easily within a few minutes to a few hours. If reactions are intense, speaking with a practitioner familiar with them is most helpful. Otherwise, one may stop a sauna program, believing it does not work or that one is becoming worse. Rarely, however, is this the case in our experience.

In the chronically ill, reactions may resolve slower as less energy is available for healing. When properly nourished and supported, however, the healing power of the body is great. It is possible, however, that reactions are not due to healing and indicate a worsening of a health condition. This usually occurs when one is not following the diet, lifestyle and other aspects of a complete healing regimen. They may also occur if one is terminally ill.

Distinguishing Healing From Disease Reactions

It is important to know if a reaction is due to healing or a worsening of a condition. Answering five questions can help one to know which is occurring.

1. Was the person following the entire health program including diet, rest, proper supplementation and the correct use of the sauna? Healing reactions most often occur when the body is given all that it requires. If the healing program is not followed strictly, the reaction is less likely due to healing.

2. Was the person feeling better before the reaction occurred? Healing reactions require energy. One's energy level often increases on a healing program until it is sufficient to initiate a reaction. Often a reaction occurs just when one is feeling stronger. If one had been feeling worse, the reaction is less likely due to healing.

3. Did the symptom ever occur in the past? Often, old symptoms or conditions recur during healing reactions. If one experienced the symptom in even the distant past, it is more likely, though not always, due to healing. One could, for example, have an aggravation of a chronic condition due to stress, fatigue or a worsening of the person's health.

4. Are the symptoms unusual? Healing reactions often produce odd or mixed symptom pictures. One may develop a sore throat or flu without fatigue, for example. It is not uncommon to have partial symptoms of an illness, since one is not really ill in the same way as if one had the full-blown condition.

5. How long have symptoms lasted? Healing reactions usually do not last long. They may be vigorous but end in a few hours or at most a week or so. If a reaction or flare-up lasts more than several weeks, it is less likely to be a healing reaction. The exception is when retracing a very chronic or deep-seated condition. This could take several weeks to several months.

Emotional Reactions

These reactions are among the most interesting and distressing at times. Anyone undergoing a sauna healing program needs to be prepared for emotional shifts as body chemistry changes, which in turn affects the brain centers. Causes of these changes include the elimination of toxins that affect the brain, changes in nutrient levels that in turn affect neurotransmitter levels, as well as general improvements in memory, cognition and clarity of thought. Other mechanisms involve returning to earlier states of body chemistry that are associated with specific emotional states or traumas. This is truly a retracing of an event that previously could not be accessed or processed completely. Following are more details regarding some of the mechanisms of emotional healing reactions.

Physically-linked Reactions. Some emotional reactions are linked to physical toxins and impaired body chemistry. An unhealthy body sends negative messages to the brain. These may be experienced as feelings of fear, anxiety or unworthiness.

Toxic metals can directly affect neurotransmitters and parts of the brain associated with anger, fear and other emotions. Iron, for example, is known to settle in the amygdala, an area of the brain associated with anger. As physical toxins are eliminated, emotional states will change. As health improves, the body sends positive messages to the brain. An emotional crisis may occur as the mind and emotional body let go of negative feelings and beliefs.

Rebalancing/Energetic Reactions. Though often not taught in psychology, *energy is required to feel feelings, even to feel depression.* Many times, a mineral analysis has revealed a pattern associated with depression. The client, however, may deny the feeling. After a time, perhaps weeks or months, the client may feel more depressed for a while, and blame their sauna therapy healing program for causing feelings of depression.

In fact, the healing program merely enhanced the client's energy and awareness. The client began to feel what had previously been inaccessible or suppressed due to a lack of energy. Once the feelings surface, they usually resolve quickly on their own.

The brain, like the body, is self-healing provided it functions correctly and is given the nutrients and other factors it requires for healing. For a psychological view of this phenomenon, I recommend Arthur Janov's *The Primal Scream* and *The Primal Revolution.*

Enhanced energy due to the elimination of toxins, improved circulation and other natural approaches, improves brain function. Clarity of thinking, memory and awareness often improve. This assists one to question beliefs about oneself and about the world. More capable of understanding oneself, false beliefs and destructive behaviors shift and may disappear altogether.

Completion Reactions. Incompletely healed mental, emotional or physical traumas often leave emotional residues. Small children often cry hard when they fall down. They 'work through' the trauma in ten minutes or so and soon are laughing as if nothing happened. This is the proper way to handle a trauma. If energy is low or if the processing of the trauma is interrupted for some other reason, a residue of the experience remains and one often develops fears or other neuroses. As energy and cognition improve, one often spontaneously heals residues of unhealed traumas.

Decompensation Reactions. Some fears and other negative attitudes and behaviors are in fact compensations for ill health or low energy. As health improves, these are no longer needed and may disappear suddenly. A surprising shift may occur, often accompanied by an insight about oneself or about the world.

Sometimes an emotional imbalance is a major stumbling block that stops the healing process until the person is willing to address it. Psychotherapy, Callahan techniques or other healing modalities may be required. Bodywork and other therapies can also be excellent to work with emotional wounds that impair the healing process.

Handling Physical Healing Reactions

In general, the body will not undertake a healing reaction unless it can see it through to completion. The most important step to take is to offer supportive measures to allow the reaction to proceed with minimal interference.

At times, one may be able to speed up a reaction so it will end sooner with natural therapies such as foot reflexology, chiropractic or other methods. Other times, one may slow down a reaction to lessen the severity of symptoms by temporarily stopping the sauna therapy for a few days. Here are general supportive instructions for healing reactions:

1. Vary the sauna sessions. Continuing with long sauna sessions can intensify a healing reaction. If the liver is being overloaded with toxins to eliminate, for example, this may not be desirable. If you suspect this, skip a few sauna sessions or reduce the frequency and/or duration of sessions until the reaction passes. However, do not let this deter you from sticking with the program. Support and encouragement are often all you need during healing reactions. Please reach out and get the support you need. Remember, you are on your way to a healthier you.

For clearing an old infection, or healing a wound or old injury that has flared up, it is often best to continue and even increase the number of sauna sessions daily to speed up the healing.

However, as a general rule, during a healing reaction, 10-15-minute sauna sessions five to eight times per day are better than long sessions. Short sessions are less debilitating in the midst of a healing reaction. If you are confused, call and speak with someone familiar with sauna therapy and healing reactions.

2. Rest lying down as much as possible. Reduce stress and strain as much as possible.. Conserve energy for healing. If possible, reduce all mental as well as physical activity. Remembering to breathe deeply and slowly is very calming for the nervous system.

3. Eat lightly. Digestion is an extra stress during healing reactions. If one is very uncomfortable, it may be best to skip a meal. One may notice that symptoms subside after eating a meal. The meal is not making one better. Energy must be diverted from healing to digest the meal, so symptoms temporarily diminish while one digests.

Drinking ample amounts of good quality distilled water is important during healing reactions. Often, drinking small amounts at a time is preferable to guzzling large glasses of water if your system is delicate.

4. Discontinue most nutritional supplements until a reaction passes. Reactions will usually proceed without most nutritional supplements. Some can impair the healing process. See the next section below for exceptions to this rule.

5. Other detoxification procedures are often helpful. Besides more frequent, shorter sauna sessions, other procedures include coffee enemas, colonic irrigation, massage, chiropractic, energy work, bodywork, foot reflexology, acupuncture and other therapies offered by competent professionals. For example, enemas are excellent and at times essential if one feels constipated or toxic. Chiropractic may help a lot when structural changes occur.

6. Call someone familiar with healing reactions if one is unsure how to handle them. Several people visited emergency rooms instead of calling me when they experienced healing reactions. They wasted hundreds of dollars and received no benefit. Those that have stayed in touch passed through healing reactions, some very vigorous, without needing medical treatment.

7. Use care when discussing healing reactions with anyone who is unfamiliar with them. Healing symptoms can easily be misinterpreted as illness. Unless a doctor, healer, or friend understands healing reactions, costly tests, emergency room visits and toxic medication are often recommended. This is a common and important problem. Medication can complicate reactions and is rarely effective. Reactions will usually proceed in spite of it. Only call someone who understands healing reactions due to sauna therapy.

Specific Supportive Measures

For Detoxification Reactions in General: As toxins are mobilized and eliminated, one may experience headaches, rashes, pain, dizziness, abdominal discomfort or other symptoms. Continuing with shorter sauna sessions usually helps symptoms pass quickly.

If a symptom persists, be sure to rest lying down a lot. This is often amazingly helpful. An excellent simple procedure to help move energy in the body's meridians is to rub the feet, including the toes, heels, ankles and the top of the foot as well as the entire bottom of the foot.

Products that may be helpful include ox bile, dehydrocholic acid and/or silymarin to enhance liver detoxification. Coffee enemas or colonic irrigation can be excellent to enhance elimination through the liver and colon. One can do up to three coffee enemas or one colon hydrotherapy session daily. One can induce vomiting if extreme nausea is present. Drink a glass of mild salt water solution first, so the stomach is not empty.

For Flare-ups of Infections: Common sites of chronic infections include the sinuses, ears, eyes, throat, bronchial tubes, lungs, intestines, kidneys and bladder. Infections may flare up as toxins are removed and as healing proceeds.

Heat activates the immune system and disables microorganisms. Symptom flare-up is desirable and if mild requires no special attention other than extra rest. Symptoms will pass in a few hours to a few weeks for very chronic infections.

If using an infrared lamp sauna, one may expose the infected area to more intense infrared as this may speed healing. Eat lightly and rest lying down as much as possible. For infections, an excellent natural remedy is bee propolis, in either a tincture, tablets or capsules. Take about 50-75 drops three times daily of a standardized extract or about 6-9 tablets or capsules daily. The tincture is thick and stains the teeth, so one can buy empty capsules and fill them with the drops as needed.

Other supplements that may be helpful include zinc, vitamin A, vitamin C, Echinacea, golden seal, lomatium, astralagus or high-quality colloidal silver. Herbs and silver may be slightly toxic, but are often less so than antibiotics.

Any infection that persists for several weeks or more may not be a healing reaction. If in doubt, always consult a knowledgeable health practitioner, as infections can become serious threats to health.

For Pain in the Liver or Kidney Area: For pain in the area of the liver, take extra ox bile, pancreatin and dehydrocholic acid (GB-3 is listed in Resources) or silymarin (milk thistle) up to 50 drops three times a day or up to 3 capsules three times per day of a standardized product. Coffee enemas may also be helpful for discomfort in the area of the liver. Occasionally, a gall bladder flush or castor oil packs may be more helpful. Basic instructions for this are on our web site, *www.drlwilson.com,* on the page entitled "Detoxification Procedures".

For pain in the kidneys or ureters, drink extra distilled water, up to one quart extra per day. Nettles, uva ursi and some kidney herbal formulas may be helpful as well.

For Diarrhea: Elimination of antibiotics, metals or toxic chemicals may cause diarrhea. Rest plenty and eat lightly. Up to six charcoal tablets, three times per day will help absorb toxins. Bioculture 3000 (Lactobacillus plantarum) from BioEnergy Systems (listed in Resources) or other lactobacillus organisms, at least three capsules, three times daily, may be helpful. Lactobacillus plantarum is the only probiotic I am aware of that helps digest proteins. This makes it most helpful for many types of parasitic infections. Some of this strain is found in Primal Defense™ and PB-8™, two popular products, but it is mixed with many others that dilute its potency. Grapefruit seed extract, olive leaf extract or high-quality colloidal silver may also help with intestinal infections.

Well-cooked garlic, 15 garlic capsules daily or Bioculture 3000 may be needed if one is releasing parasites. Eat lightly of non-fibrous, non-irritating foods such as rice, other grains, chicken and vegetable soup until diarrhea passes. Severe diarrhea that persists requires further intervention. Otherwise one may lose vital electrolytes and become dehydrated.

For Emotional Reactions: Emotional traumas deeply held need to be brought to consciousness to be released. When emotions or negative thoughts arise, allow oneself to feel them without suppressing them or wallowing in the feelings. Observe feelings from as neutral a viewpoint as possible. It is very helpful to talk with someone supportive to gain added perspective. Feelings will generally pass, washing over oneself like ocean waves. The Observation-Meditation Exercise taught by Roy Masters may be very helpful. (See www.drlwilson.com or the Foundation of Human Understanding, www.fhu.org). Vigorous exercise can slow emotional reactions. Extra rest and sleep will help them pass more quickly.

Many people learned well to suppress their feelings and have great difficulty expressing them. One may become afraid of one's own buried feelings. Allow oneself to cry, scream or otherwise express that which you feel. If this seems embarrassing, one can close the bedroom door or go sit in a car. For several years I would cry for no apparent reason, often in crowded places. At times I believed I was ill, but eventually the symptom passed and I found myself much happier.

For Nervousness And Anxiety: The elimination of stored caffeine, theophylline, diet pills or other stimulant substances can cause temporary feelings of anxiety as they are released. These will pass without requiring supportive therapy. Extreme fatigue or copper elimination can also cause feelings of anxiety.

If a feeling is very intense or persistent, nutritional supplements of calcium, magnesium, zinc, GABA or choline may have a calming effect. Liquid supplements, or grinding or chewing tablets will provide a faster effect. One may take up to 2500 mg of calcium, 1500 mg of magnesium, 100 mg of zinc, 1500 mg of GABA and/or 800 mg of choline in a 24-hour period.

Resting, deep, slow breathing, taking a walk, calming herbs, homeopathic remedies, massage, foot reflexology and other natural therapies may be helpful as well.

To Slow Healing Reactions: Choline, 100 mg 3 times per day, will help slow the elimination of toxic metals and chemicals. Aspirin, Tylenol, tranquilizers or other over-the-counter remedies are less recommended.

For Weight Loss or Gain: During sauna therapy, weight will often fluctuate. Weight gain may occur if the body retains water to buffer toxins that are being eliminated. Weight loss may occur even in a thin person as poor quality tissue is broken down. One often will go through periods of greater tissue breakdown followed by periods of rebuilding. Shifts in glandular activity may temporarily cause weight gain or loss.

Most shifts in weight are not a cause for concern. In a few cases, eating more or fewer calories may assist in balancing weight during a detoxification program. Usually, however, the therapy program needs to take its course and weight will normalize after several months to a year or more, depending on the toxicity of the body.

Discussing Healing Reactions

Forewarned, most people handle healing reactions well. One should look forward to reactions as they are evidence of deep healing. However, they often catch one off guard, coming at a time when one is feeling significantly better. They can also affect one's judgment, causing doubt and fear.

For this reason, *always call someone knowledgeable if needed when a reaction occurs*, so that therapy can be modified. Those who stay in touch fare best on sauna therapy programs. Otherwise one may stop the program prematurely or end up in a hospital when this is usually unnecessary and not helpful. Often, drugs and other remedies are not too effective during a healing reaction because the body wants to go through the reaction, and because one is not 'ill' in the usual sense of the word during a healing reaction.

These guidelines are sufficient to handle most healing reactions. I have worked with over 50,000 clients as a nutrition consultant. Healing reactions with a nutritional balancing program can be vigorous, but are rarely dangerous because the program tends to balance the body so well. So far, I have never required medical intervention for a healing reaction during a nutritional balancing program, provided the person follows the program correctly. *However, always use common sense and do not hesitate to seek help if you are not sure what to do.*

12
Sauna Design

"I am 65 years old. For the first time since I was 18 I have energy again to go places and do things. Since the age of 16 I worked in the construction of oil refineries and was exposed to many paints, solvents, refinery wastes and metals. I became tired, felt boxed in, did not want to communicate and was often constipated with gas and bloating.

Several years ago I visited a metabolic clinic in Mexico where I got some relief with hydrogen peroxide baths, enemas and many supplements. However, it did not last. I have used an infrared lamp sauna every day for a year and my energy level is finally consistently better. - Mr. J.H., Houston, TX

Saunas consist of two main parts, an enclosure and a heat source. Let us begin by discussing various ways to heat a sauna.

Heat Sources

Heat is generated by vibrating molecules at a rapid rate. These molecules may be of water, air or some other substance. Once heat is created, it must be transferred to the sauna bather unless he or she is heated directly by radiant heating. Saunas may use radiant heating, or two other methods to transfer heat to the sauna bather. *Convection* occurs when warm air moves around the body. *Conduction* involves heating the body by direct contact, such as a heating pad, steam or hot water.

Radiant heating involves the use of infrared energy. Infrared is a heat-emitting spectrum of frequencies between 0.5 and 1000 microns (or micrometers) or 500 to 1,000,000 nanometers. Infrared is divided roughly into near, middle and far infrared frequencies. *Near infrared* is about 0.5 to 1.7 microns, *middle infrared* is about 1.7 to 4 microns and *far infrared* 4 to 1000 microns. Infrared vibrates the water molecules inside objects. The sun heats by the radiant method.

Convection Saunas

Traditional saunas heat the bather by moving hot air. In olden times saunas used wood fires while modern ones usually employ gas or electric heaters. Rocks heated in a fire heat

Native American sweat lodges. Rocks are heated outside and carried into the sweat lodge. Heated rocks heat up the air and emit a little infrared energy as well.

A wood fire within a sauna is smoky and may deplete oxygen. Wood, gas or electric stoves or heaters are much cleaner. Hot rocks work well but require preparation to build the fire and transport the rocks inside. Most hot air saunas use gas or electric coil heaters. Connected to thermostats and timers, they are clean and simple to operate. Electric heaters often have a few rocks on top of the heater so bathers can sprinkle water on them to produce steam.

Radiant Heating

Infrared and far infrared saunas are heated by the radiant method. This is important due to the special benefits of radiant heating:

- It is highly efficient, so these saunas use much less electricity and require little if any preheating.
- It penetrates the skin and heats from inside as well as on the skin. This helps the heat reach deeper tissues.
- It does not heat the air, so the ambient temperature remains lower and more comfortable for many people.
- It is highly compatible with the human body, which assists detoxification and healing.

Infrared Sauna Disadvantages. Infrared heaters do not allow one to make steam in the sauna. Also, seating arrangements may be less flexible in an infrared sauna. For maximum benefits, one needs to position oneself directly in the path of the radiant energy. One can wear light clothing in a hot air sauna. It is less recommended in an infrared sauna as it blocks some of the rays. Dark-colored clothing could also possibly ignite if it became hot enough.

Two Types Of Infrared Saunas

Two types of infrared saunas are available. The *far infrared* type employs six to twelve ceramic or metallic elements that emit mainly in a narrow band of energy in the far infrared range, usually between about 4 and 40 microns. The heating elements are built into several walls of the sauna so the rays strike all parts of the body for direct radiant heating.

The other type uses *infrared heat lamps* to heat the occupants. The first infrared lamp sauna was constructed by John Harvey Kellogg, MD in 1891. It worked extremely well, although it used regular incandescent bulbs that gave off a lot of light as well. It never caught on in America. However, Dr. Kellogg sold many in Europe, including to European royalty. The original units used 40 small incandescent bulbs placed around the enclosure. Infrared lamps and far infrared emitters had not been invented.

A modern one-person infrared lamp sauna uses three or four 250-watt, reddish, infrared heat lamps. These are easily available for purchase at hardware stores. These lamps emit yellow, orange and red light as well as mostly near infrared energy. They also emit some middle infrared and a little far infrared energy. The next chapter discusses many technical aspects about them as well as design considerations. Halogen heat lamps are also available. However, I do not recommend them as their spectrum does not appear to be as healthful.

Hot Sand or Solar Power

Professor Serge Jurasunas of Portugal developed an interesting type of sauna therapy using a special sand from Japan that emits infrared in the range of 4-14 microns. Heating occurs by direct contact of the body with the hot sand. He claims excellent results with pesticide elimination, cancer and other conditions. This therapy is described in an article in the *Townsend Letter*, 203:123-134, June 2000.

Solar energy could be used for sauna heating with the proper setup. However, it would only work at certain hours and temperature control might be difficult. The following chart summarizes the methods of heating saunas:

Mainly Radiant Heating:	Infrared lamp sauna
	Far infrared sauna
	Solar sauna
Mainly Convection Heating:	Electric coil heater, hot rocks
	Fire inside the sauna
	Wood or gas stove heater
Conduction Heating:	Infrared-emitting sand

Electromagnetic Fields

Disruptive electromagnetic (EM) fields may not be an important issue if one is only using a sauna occasionally. They can be important, however, when a sauna is used daily for therapy. Electric heaters in hot air saunas produce weak electromagnetic fields. These do not interfere with therapy for most people. Gas heaters, wood stoves or heating with hot rocks produce no EM emissions.

Far infrared saunas can produce significant disruptive EM fields. One company claims to shield their far infrared sauna to reduce EM emissions. Infrared lamp saunas produce no detectable EM fields.

Cabinets and Enclosures

Most saunas encompass the entire body in which one either sits or lies down. An alternative is a *sauna cabinet* resembling a steam cabinet. In this case, the head is not exposed to the heat. However, heating the sinuses, ears and nasal passages is beneficial. A cabinet may be more comfortable but will be less effective. It can be used for those who are very claustrophobic or those who have difficulty breathing in a sauna.

A third option for those who are bedridden is to warm up an entire bedroom or a part of a bedroom that has been partitioned off with a curtain or other method. This is most feasible with an infrared lamp sauna as it operates at a lower temperature and just requires several heat lamps that can be positioned over the bed or off to one side. Since it only pertains to lamp saunas, this option is discussed in more detail in the next chapter.

Materials

Finnish-style saunas are of masonry and/or wood, often cedar or poplar. Tongue-and-groove boards avoid nails or glue that may react to extreme heat and moisture. High-end saunas feature beautiful woodwork and design. Saunas made of cedar may outgas terpenes. Manufacturers may kiln-dry cedar to reduce or avoid outgassing. Modern saunas may also be made of poplar, fir or even mostly glass to avoid outgassing. Sauna cabinets may be made of wood, fabric, vinyl or ABS plastic.

Native American sweat lodges are made of branches tied to form a dome-shaped frame. Blankets or animal hides cover the frame.

Insulation

If constructing a sauna outside, double-wall construction or some kind of insulation will be required in cold climates. Fiberglass, cellulose insulation or thick wood would be fine. Reflectix, a thin aluminum-coated sandwich material with plastic bubbles in between, may be used. Styrofoam may outgas into the sauna unless a barrier is placed between the foam and the interior wall of the sauna. Tar paper as a barrier may outgas. Corrugated cardboard is a fair insulator and inexpensive. I do not recommend aluminum material inside a sauna.

The outside of an outdoor sauna may be painted, but not the inside as it will outgas. One may also shingle the outside, add stucco or an exterior siding material for protection against the elements.

Inside a home at room temperature, insulation is less important. 1/4" to 3/4"-thick 2x6 boards, wood siding, plywood or even masonite should provide adequate insulation. Even double-thickness canvas or other medium-weight fabric is adequate in a warm room to insulate a sauna.

Size

Saunas range from one-person models to large public sauna rooms. Partial-body cabinets are for one person and resemble steam cabinets. They usually fit through a standard interior door opening.

Hot air saunas need some room for the heater unit. Far infrared saunas do not need extra space for the heating elements, as they are embedded in the walls of the sauna. An infrared lamp sauna needs about 9" for the lamps if they mount inside the sauna. Also, one needs room to rotate the body. This means one needs a stool, small chair or bench on which one can rotate.

Build a one-person lamp sauna enclosure about 3-4' wide by 4' long x 5'-6' high. This allows one to sit comfortably and rotate. For a two-person model, a good size is about 4' x 6-7' wide by 5-6' high. Far infrared saunas are sold that hold up to about four people.

Sauna rooms may be much larger and hold 10 or more people. These are usually hot air saunas, which are less recommended. Native American sweat lodges are often no more than four feet high and often large enough to hold 20-30 people.

Sitting, Lying or Standing Up

Seating arrangements are most flexible in a hot air sauna. One may sit upright or lie in a horizontal position anywhere in the sauna. In an infrared sauna, one needs to be directly exposed to the rays. This usually means sitting upright in a designated location, although one may lie down as well.

The best body position for therapy is seated unless one is unable to sit. One will tend to sweat the most in this position and in an infrared lamp sauna it is easiest to adjust one's distance from the infrared heat lamps in the seated position. Also when seated, the head gets hotter as it is higher up in the sauna. This is beneficial as it promotes sweating to help remove the large amount of toxins often stored in the brain, hypothalamus, pituitary and thyroid glands. Rarely, a person has difficulty tolerating the heat on the head.

Some prefer lying down for comfort or because one cannot sit for 30-40 minutes at a time. Far infrared saunas may not work quite as well lying down, as less of the body is in the direct line of the ceramic elements.

If one wishes to lie down in an infrared lamp sauna, lamps can be placed on the ceiling of the sauna. Make sure the distance from the body to the lamps is 18" to 30". One must turn over frequently to expose the entire body to the infrared rays. *Be sure to place a piece of metal window screen inside the wire lamp guard if you are lying down with the lamps above you.* This will protect you in the rare event that a lamp should break.

Standing up for sauna therapy is not recommended. The effort required does not permit as much inhibition of the sympathetic nervous system.

Shape

Most full-body sauna enclosures are rectangular boxes. Some designs are hexagonal, octagonal or even circular. Traditional sweat lodges are dome-shaped. This is a perfect shape for a convection sauna. The shape promotes even heating, allowing one to sit anywhere and receive the benefits. The dome is also highly efficient. It requires up to one fourth less material to construct than a rectangle and has the least surface area through which heat can be lost.

Saunas often have a ceiling less than 6' high to keep the heat near the bathers. In large saunas, the higher up one sits, the more intense the heat.

Portability

If portability is an issue, sauna cabinets and small full-body enclosures are designed to be easily moved. Smaller enclosures are often constructed of panels that fasten together quickly. Infrared lamp saunas may be built to be very portable. Frame saunas and those installed in existing bathrooms or closets are ideal for apartments and other small dwellings. Frame sauna enclosures made of PVC pipe or thin wood are extremely lightweight.

Thermometers

Every sauna should have a thermometer. The three basic types are digital (electronic), bimetallic (springy metal) and liquid-filled. Digital and bimetallic are the most accurate. Liquid-filled may be less accurate, though quality varies. For infrared lamp saunas, an inexpensive outdoor thermometer that reads to 120° F should be adequate. Manufacturers such as Saunamatic in Colorado Springs (800-472-8627) sell thermometers and other accessories for hot air saunas that read to 250° or higher.

The temperature within a sauna varies, warmer at the top than at the bottom. A hot air sauna has a more uniform temperature due to convection heating. In an infrared sauna, if possible place the thermometer out of the direct path of the infrared lamps or far infrared heaters.

Thermostats

A thermostat is a type of thermometer that is hooked up to your heat source. It turns the heat on and off depending on the temperature at which the thermostat is set. Most commercial saunas come with automatic thermostats. These are important in hot air saunas to prevent overheating. In an infrared sauna, one wants the lamps or elements to remain on at all times. It is usually best to receive the maximum exposure to the beneficial infrared energy. Thus this type of sauna is best used without a thermostat. Simply open the door slightly when the temperature reaches about 110-115° F to prevent overheating.

If your infrared sauna has a thermostat, to prevent automatic shutoff set it higher than you desire. When the temperature reaches optimum, open the door about 1/4" so the temperature does not continue to increase. This will prevent the thermostat from shutting off the lamps.

Timers

Most commercial saunas come with automatic timers. One can simply use a clock or kitchen timer, though an automatic one is a nice feature if one tends to lose track of time or might fall asleep in a sauna.

Ventilation

Sauna ventilation may be important. Openings at or near the top of a sauna clear odors, metal vapors and volatile chemicals eliminated with the sweat. Ventilation also introduces fresh air to make breathing more pleasant. Native American and other traditional sweat lodges may not provide ventilation. However, many of these are not air tight due to their construction.

Modern sauna designs are often ventilated. If one builds a sauna, one can leave a 1" by 8" opening above the door and on the opposite side as well. Some designs include a louvered opening so that ventilation can be regulated. If one builds an infrared lamp sauna in a closet or bathroom, the door may be opened slightly every five minutes if there is no other ventilation.

Ventilating the top of the sauna will not significantly reduce the temperature inside provided the rest of the enclosure is airtight. Ventilation is not required in a partial-body cabinet if the head is exposed.

Leave the door open when not using a sauna to facilitate odor removal and drying of the sauna.

Inability To Heat Up

A sauna may not heat up because 1) it may be too large and need extra heating, 2) it needs better insulating, 3) it may have air leaks, especially at the bottom of the enclosure, 4) the ceiling may be too high or 5) it is in a cold room or patio that hinders heating.

Ventilation at the top of a sauna is excellent, but air leaks at the bottom of a sauna will prevent proper heating. Closet doors and shower doors often are not airtight at the bottom. One may need to add weather stripping, stuff a towel under the door or use some other material in cracks to correct air leaks.

Bathtub enclosures used as saunas may have tile that stays cold to the touch, especially if it is on an outside wall. In a bathroom, one may need to tape cardboard or other insulating material over the tile to retain the heat. Single-pane glass used in shower stalls and other enclosures is a poor insulator and may need to be covered with cardboard, fabric or another insulating material.

If the ceiling is over six feet high, you may be able to install a false ceiling of plywood, fabric or cardboard. If the volume of the space is larger than the heating capacity of the heat source, one needs to add more heating capacity. One way is to add a small electric heater or some other source of heat. Adding another infrared lamp is another solution.

Rotting

Physicians who have heavily-used steam sauna detoxification centers report that floors of wood saunas eventually rot. Acids and other chemicals eliminated in sweat soak into the porous wood and harbor bacteria and mold that cannot be washed out. Non-porous materials such as tile, glass, fiberglass or metal do not have this problem. Rotting is less likely in an infrared sauna that does not use steam, and less likely in a home setting. Suggestions to reduce or avoid the problem in saunas that are used in the home include:

- Cover the floor completely with a large towel. Lift it up at the end of a session, letting it dry. One need not wash this towel after each session.
- If one sits on a wooden bench or stool, cover it with a small towel. Even better, cover the bench with a piece of clear vinyl and place the towel on top of the vinyl when entering the sauna. Most sweat will accumulate on the small towel.
- Wipe sweat off the body frequently with another small towel, rather than letting it drip on the floor. After the session, rinse off the two small towels in the shower until they do not smell. Wash them periodically in a washing machine.
- Do not leave wet towels, slippers or anything else on the floor of a sauna.
- Keep the sauna door open when not in use. This helps dry the sauna.
- Clean the sauna floor with Oxiclean™ or another non-toxic, odor-free product that oxidizes bacteria and mold. Apply Oxiclean™ dissolved in warm water with a sponge and wipe off any excess. Cleaning the floor once a month is probably adequate in a home sauna, depending on how much one uses the sauna. If one notices discoloration of the sauna floor, apply it more often. Oxiclean™ is also excellent to add when laundering towels used in a sauna.

13
Lamp Sauna Considerations

"I have a 64-year history of migraine headaches that began when I was 2 years old. I was incapacitated much of the time and had become addicted to Imitrex (medication).

A healthful diet and many types of therapy were only minimally helpful. Two years ago I built an infrared lamp sauna. It has been indispensable for my healing program of detoxification and balancing my body chemistry. I am excited to report that for the first time in my life I can control the headaches, rather than having them control me.

The sauna also allows me to sweat out PCPs and various other chemicals including food additives, and air and water pollutants. It also helps clear the spirit as well as the body. I have named my sauna "The Dragon", the hot fiery breath of purification." - Mr. N.P., Prescott, AZ

This chapter is essentially a brief manual about infrared lamp saunas. It answers many questions about their operation, safety and design considerations for various configurations. If this is not of interest, one may skip this chapter.

Lying Down or Sitting

In an infrared lamp sauna, body position is important as one needs to be exposed directly to the infrared rays. Also, unless the lamps are all around the enclosure, one needs to be able to rotate the body to expose all sides to the rays.

Some people prefer to lie down in a sauna, which means the lamps need to be either overhead or at one's side. This can be done, providing the bather is willing to turn over frequently to expose the whole body to the infrared rays.

A few people have built PVC pipe frame enclosures designed for lying down instead of sitting. In fact, the frame sauna enclosure described in Appendix E can be easily modified so one can lie down inside instead of sitting. Simply flip the enclosure so that the lamps sit overhead. Entry and exit issues are somewhat more complex, but can be worked out for those who cannot sit or prefer lying down for other reasons.

Here are a few cautions concerning overhead lamps:

- Add a piece of metal window screen to the lamp guard to add extra protection in case a lamp should break while a person is taking a sauna.

- Make sure the distance is correct from the end of the lamp to the bather's body. If the lamps are too close, one could receive a burn. If they are too far away, the effect will be lessened. The ideal distance from the lamps to the bather is about 24" for most people. Some people are more sensitive than others and may need to be even further from the lamps.
- One can fall asleep lying down much easier than when sitting up. Set a timer for the lamps and preferably have a friend in attendance to make sure you do not fall asleep.
- The maximum number of lamps overhead should not be greater than five.
- Do not place a lamp directly over the head unless you first read the section below entitled Cautions Regarding Aiming A Lamp Directly At The Head.

For Those Who Are Bedridden

An entire small room or part of a room may be used as a sauna enclosure for those who have difficulty being moved. A small, upstairs and well-insulated room will be easier to heat. Also, the lower the ceiling, the easier it will be to heat. For the floor or the room, carpeting is warmer than wood, which in turn is warmer than tile or cement. A ground floor room with a cement floor will be difficult to heat sufficiently for sauna therapy unless one has in-floor heating.

One option is to cordon off part of a room, similar to the way hospital rooms have curtains that can be pulled around a patient's bed for privacy. However, for this to work well, one must place a piece of fabric, cardboard, plywood or other material over the top of the enclosed area so that heat will not escape. One essentially builds a fabric sauna around the patient's bed.

If heating an entire room or part of a room, an extra space heater will usually be needed to raise the temperature to 110° F. or even a little higher. An unconventional heating method is to use a number of the reddish infrared lamps around the room, as this is an efficient method of heating. Be sure to mount them safely in sockets designed for 250-watt lamps. Protect the lamps from accidentally being touched or banged, and be sure the lamps' heat will not damage objects in the room. If you live in a warm climate, warming the room may be quite easy by opening the windows and shutting off the air conditioning.

Lamp Placement. The lamps used for therapy may be mounted above the patient's bed on a frame that is hung from the ceiling, or for safety or convenience they may be placed on one or even both sides of the bed. Lamps overhead are somewhat better as they will shine on a greater percentage of the body at one time and are out of the way of the bed.

If lamps are overhead, one arrangement is a trianglular setup with one lamp shining on the chest and two on the abdomen. An extra lamp could be placed at the feet. An alternative is to arrange four lamps in a straight line running from head to feet. A separate switch for the lamp over the head would be excellent. See the section below about aiming a lamp directly at the head.

Mount the lamps on a piece of plywood or other framing material and hang the unit carefully from the ceiling. If possible, make the height adjustable with rope or wires so that the distance from the lamps to the patient can be varied depending on the patient's condition and skin sensitivity.

If lamps are placed on one side of a bed, the best arrangement is a line of three or four lamps, with one perhaps aimed toward the head and neck, one toward the chest and one or two aimed at the abdomen and legs. *Always place guards over the lamps to prevent accidentally touching or banging a lamp..*

The patient will have to be turned every few minutes and after the session either sponged off or toweled off. Many ill people do not sweat easily and need to begin with short sessions of 10-15 minutes until they begin to sweat more easily. A rubber sheet or other moisture protection will be needed on the bed.

If building an enclosure around a bedridden patient is difficult, or if the patient is extremely debilitated, another option is simply to place one or more in infrared lamps over the patient or on one side of the bed. This will not provide as much heating, and sweating will be less. However, it offers excellent infrared benefits and may cause some local sweating as well.

Cautions Regarding Aiming A Lamp Directly At The Head

A lamp aimed directly toward the head can be beneficial. This is especially true in cases of brain fog, parasitic infections and to help remove toxic metals and chemicals from the brain, which everyone has to some degree. However, please observe the following important rules:

- If possible, wait until one has been taking regular saunas at least several times a week for five months. This is important so the body is well-acclimated to the sauna. The exception is a serious brain condition such as a tumor or parasitic infection that requires immediate aggressive intervention. I recommend close medical supervision in this case, and begin with only five minutes with the lamp on the head to gauge the body's reaction.
- Use only one 250-watt lamp. If one can locate a 150-watt lamp, it would be better in some cases.
- The overhead lamp must be 24 " or more from the head.
- This procedure is generally best for slow oxidizers. These are people with a tendency for sluggish thyroid and adrenal glandular activity. If one is hyperthyroid, or you suspect a fast metabolic rate, use more caution.
- Remain in a sauna with an lamp at the head no more than 40 minutes daily.
- Turn off the lamps and leave the sauna if one feels very nauseous or dizzy.
- A lamp aimed at the head is never a substitute for lamps that shine directly on the chest and abdomen.
- A separate switch to control this lamp is most helpful.

Lamps To Warm The Legs

The lower part of any sauna is much cooler than the upper part. Some people notice their legs sweat less than the rest of their body for this reason.

The most critical organs to reach with the infrared rays are those of the body trunk. As overall health improves, most conditions of the extremities will improve.

However, an extra lamp at the level of the legs can enhance the sauna experience and may help heal conditions affecting the legs much faster. An extra lamp at this level will also speed up the heating of the sauna. *It is critical to place a guard over this lamp,* as it is very easy to kick it with your feet. Also, a separate switch to control the lower lamp is helpful to keep the sauna from becoming too hot. Be sure the lamp cord can handle the total wattage for all the lamps.

Guards For Lamps

One must place a guard in front of infrared heat lamps. These lamps are both very hot and somewhat delicate. They often last several years and are inexpensive to replace. However, they can shatter if hit hard enough, or rarely one breaks for no apparent reason. This is discussed in a later section.

The simplest guard is a piece of wire mesh, also called hardware cloth, bent to fit around the lamps and fastened to the enclosure. Welded wire or steel or brass rods could also be bent to fit around the lamps. Some portable lamp sockets used for brood lights come with aluminum reflectors and steel guards in front of the lamps. Aluminum is less recommended inside a sauna, as some may volatilize and one could breathe the fumes. Older portable lamp sockets used steel reflectors, which are preferable.

Another alternative is to recess the lamps in 'cans' used for home lighting. Be sure to order special ones designed for 250-watt bulbs. Recessing lamps so they are actually outside the sauna is safer and frees up space within the enclosure. This means the enclosure can be smaller, or if it is the same size, it will be roomier.

The only problem with recessing lamps is that one would like to capture as much of the heat as possible from the lamps to heat the enclosure. If the lamps are outside the enclosure, heat may be lost to the outside atmosphere.

Multiple-Person Lamp saunas

A two-person infrared lamp sauna requires two or three extra lamps. Ideally, these should be placed on the same wall as the first three lamps next to the others. This way two can sit side by side. The enclosure needs to be two to three feet wider to accommodate a second bather.

Wire the extra lamps with a separate switch. This way, if only one person is using the sauna, the sole bather would only switch on three of the lamps. However, due to the larger enclosure, one may need to switch on all the lamps to heat up the space and then turn off the extra ones once the sauna heats up. I do not recommend aiming more than four or five 250-watt infrared lamps toward oneself at any time. Another option is to use a small space heater to help heat a larger space.

In theory, an infrared lamp sauna can be built for any number of bathers. The principle to recall is to set up the seating arrangement so that the rays can reach on every bather.

Why Lamps On Only One Wall?

At times in this book, lamps are recommended on only one wall. Reasons for this are:

- *More focused energy.* With all three lamps on one wall, energy can be focused more powerfully on one area of the body than if the lamps are on several walls.
- *Ease of construction and permitting a smaller enclosure.* Since the lamps may extend into the enclosure, if they are placed on several walls one needs a larger enclosure to allow room for them. This would not be the case if the lamps are recessed. In this case, however, the lamp sockets must extend outside the sauna.
- *Enhanced circulatory effects.* With lamps on one wall, one must rotate to heat all sides of the body. This causes blood to move from one side of the body to another throughout the session, somewhat enhancing the sauna's circulatory effects.
- *Safety.* With lamps on only one wall, it is easier to remember where they are at all time, which helps avoid accidentally bumping or touching a hot lamp.

A number of people have built units with lamps on two walls and report doing well with this arrangement. I do not recommend using more than four or five 250-watt infrared lamps on one person at a time.

Converting A Sauna Or Steam Cabinet

One can convert a hot air sauna or a far infrared sauna to an infrared lamp sauna. First, ascertain there is access to about 7 amps of electric power to operate three 250-watt infrared lamps. Also be sure one can sit between 18" and 24" from where infrared lamps will be placed. This generally requires that the sauna be at least four feet long on one side. Also, one will need to rotate the body to expose all parts to the rays. Many saunas have fixed benches on one side. However, they are often easy to remove and replace with a stool or bench in the middle to allow free rotation. One could use the existing bench, but rotation may be more difficult this way.

If the sauna to be converted is larger than about 4' x 4' or taller than 6', leave the original heater in place as it will be needed to help heat the sauna. Add several infrared lamps in the configuration shown in Appendix D. If the sauna to be converted is smaller than about 4' x 4', one may remove the old heater if desired as the heat lamps should suffice for heating.

Converting a steam cabinet to a lamp sauna or adding lamps to a steam cabinet is difficult because the cabinets are usually too small to allow one to sit about two feet from the lamps. Also, it is difficult to turn around in the cabinet. Also, one should not allow water vapor to touch the lamps as this can cause a fire hazard.

Other Design Considerations

Brands of Lamps. To the best of my knowledge, all the popular brands of lamps have very similar technical specifications and all are acceptable for therapy. Red (or reddish) infrared lamps emit a wide spectrum of frequencies. According to data supplied by Osram Sylvania, in the visible spectrum the lamps emit a small amount of yellow and significantly more orange and red light. In the infrared spectrum, the output peaks in the near infrared range, about 1200 nanometers or 1.2 microns. However, they also emit significantly in the middle infrared and some in the far infrared range. The lamps' filaments are covered with red glass so they emit very little green, blue, violet or ultraviolet radiation. A graph of their spectral power distribution is at the end of this chapter.

I recommend Havel-SLi, GE, Philips, Sylvania, Halco or Feit brands of *250-watt heat lamps.* Most do not say 'infrared' on the label. They cost about $8-15 US dollars each. As of this printing (2014), Westinghouse is coating their lamps with Teflon that outgases a little. I do not recommend clear heat lamps or any other type of lamps.

Enclosure Materials. The best materials for lamp sauna enclosures include wood, metal, glass, Reflectix, or a natural fabric. Less recommended materials include fiberglass, laminated wood, particle board, masonite, plastics and synthetic fabrics. These materials will outgas to some degree and are definitely unsuitable for anyone sensitive to chemicals.

However, the outgassing problem is less critical in an infrared lamp sauna because it operates at a relatively low temperature. For example, plywood, masonite or other laminate materials can work well unless one is chemically sensitive to the glue they contain. Plexiglass may be used for a window or even part of a wall or two. This is helpful for those who are claustrophobic. Glass reflects infrared energy, but is a poor insulator.

Frames And Other Low-Cost Designs. Lamp saunas need not be of wood. A low-cost, portable design is to build a frame made of wood, metal or PVC pipe. Install an electric light unit inside and hang blankets or fabric over the frame to cover it. This can form an excellent simple enclosure.

At the time of this printing, we sell a unit of this design. You may build one from the plans in Appendix E if you are handy, and save about $100-200.00. Be sure to place lamps away from any flammable material. Also, do not leave the unit on when you are not present.

A woman wrote the author that she built an infrared lamp sauna in which the floor and one wall of her enclosure were made of pine boards screwed to a 2" x 2" frame. The lamp sockets were placed on the wooden wall. The rest of the enclosure consisted of a 2" x 2" frame with cardboard from refrigerator boxes stapled to the wood frame. The best arrangement would be a double thickness construction as cardboard is only a fair insulator. It may also outgas a little, particularly if it is new. In this design, the door fit between two extra vertical 2" x 2"s. The doorframe was of 1" x 4" wood with cardboard stapled to both sides. The door had a small stained glass window in it. Total cost for the sauna was under $200.00.

Another woman wrote that she mounted four red infrared lamps in her bathroom in the correct configuration, along with using a room heater to heat up the bathroom. She claims this was sufficient to achieve the correct temperature. This will only work in a very small bathroom with a low ceiling.

Cross Bars. Some wooden saunas come with horizontal rails made of 2" x 2" running the length of the sauna on each side, about 3 feet from the floor. Although not necessary, I find these most helpful to hold on to when one gets up or rotates inside the sauna. They also stiffen the structure.

Handicap Modification. If a lamp sauna is to be used by someone in a wheelchair or on crutches, horizontal cross bars described above may be very helpful. The enclosure needs to be about 4' x 5' or wider to allow room to rotate.

To hold the heat in a larger lamp sauna enclosure, one may make the ceiling lower, add a small electric heater to assist heating or add an extra lamp. A rotating stool may be easier to sit on for some handicapped people than a conventional bench that does not rotate.

If using a regular wheelchair, the seat back of the chair will interfere with the healing effects by blocking infrared radiation. It may be possible to remove the back and replace it with nylon cord, or wood or plastic ribbing so that the person's back is exposed to the heat and infrared energy.

A convenient on-off switch is important for a handicapped person and the thermometer and timer should be easy to read. Time in the sauna should be reduced if one is debilitated. Also, metallic parts of wheelchairs and crutches, especially if dark-colored, may heat up excessively in an infrared sauna. Avoid touching them or wrap electrical tape around them.

Bathroom And Closet Installation

Small Closets And Small Bathrooms. These can make excellent lamp sauna enclosures. If using a closet or other small room, here are some considerations:

- Small air leaks at the top of the door of a closet or bathroom are acceptable. Air leaks at the bottom may impair the heating of the sauna. One can add weather stripping to seal the leaks, or perhaps position a towel to seal the bottom of a door.
- An extra heater may be needed if the room is larger than about four feet by four feet.
- Lowering the ceiling to four or five feet in a closet or bathroom will assist heating. One may do this with a piece of plywood, or even cardboard or fabric nailed to the walls. The false ceiling need not be totally airtight.
- A lamp unit can be hung on a bathroom door or even from a towel rack. Always be sure to have guards on the lamps and move slowly and cautiously in the room.

Bathtubs And Shower Stalls. These can also make acceptable lamp sauna enclosures, especially if the bathtub is not used for bathing. Here are some considerations for tub enclosures:

- Do not allow water to get on or near the infrared lamps.
- You must close in the top of the tub area so heat will not escape.
- If you have no other space for a sauna and must use the tub for bathing, hang the light unit in such a way that you can either remove it for showering or cover it well to avoid getting it wet.
- *Be sure to unplug the electrical unit before bathing near it.*
- Tile and glass used in tub areas are poor insulators and often cold. This may prevent a sauna from heating up sufficiently. A sauna should heat up to 110° F within about 30-40 minutes. If it does not, check for air leaks at the bottom or add insulation by placing fabric or corrugated cardboard over tile, glass or other cold surfaces.
- Vinyl shower curtains are fair insulators. You may substitute a fabric curtain or double the thickness by adding a second vinyl curtain. Be sure to keep plastic or fabric curtains away from the hot lamps.

- Glass or plastic tub doors are often not airtight on the bottom. To heat up properly, a sauna requires a fairly airtight door on the bottom. One may push a towel under the door or use tape over the opening to plug air leaks.
- Small, square shower stalls are usually not large enough for an infrared lamp sauna, as the space required is at least 3' x 4'. That is, *one wall of the enclosure must be about four feet long. Otherwise, you will be sitting too close to the lamps.* The only ways around this problem are to recess the lamps into one wall if possible or find less powerful lamps. I have not seen lower wattage red heat lamps in hardware stores. However, they are manufactured here or abroad and may become available.

Lamp Safety

Sylvania supplied a safety rating for 250R40 red infrared lamps. They are extremely safe because they emit very little ultraviolet. The latter can cause cataracts, skin cancer and aging of the skin. In fact, infrared is an antidote for sun damage due to ultraviolet rays.

Some temporary reddening of the skin often occurs in a far infrared or infrared lamp sauna. This will disappear in less than an hour. Regarding burns from the heat, according to Dr. Robert Levin, research engineer at Sylvania and an expert on infrared, one will feel the heat and the burn before any tissue damage can occur.

The following incidents have been reported to me: A burn occurred in a patient with a large skin graft on his arm. The area has no sensation of heat. He placed his arm near an infrared lamp and left it there too long as he felt no heat from it. This resulted in a few blisters on the arm. Another slight burn occurred when a patient rubbed essential oil of oregano on his face and then went into the sauna. This also caused some blistering. It is unclear whether the burn was due to the lamps or just to the oil, which is very irritating. *Never put oils on the skin before entering an infrared or far infrared sauna.*

If a person is very sensitive to the heat or light, I recommend unscrewing one of the heat lamps. Another option is to place a piece of metal window screen inside the lamp guard, which will reduce the intensity of the heat and light.

Lamp Breakage

Infrared heat lamps can break if bumped hard enough. Rarely one even shatters just when turned on. This is unfortunate and indicates a need for better manufacturing control.

I am aware of three occasions out of some 500 reports from those who are using lamp saunas in which a lamp broke while in use. One case involved a Feit brand of lamp. The person accidentally threw some water on the hot lamp. A second involved a Philips lamp, and no obvious reason for breakage was given. The third I have no information about, as it was reported to me second-hand. One person received superficial cuts when a lamp shattered. I am not aware of any serious injuries at this time.

For obvious safety reasons, *a guard in front of the lamps is essential.* Also, if you set up an infrared lamp sauna with the lamps above the bather or if very concerned about lamp breakage, install a piece of metal window screen inside of the lamp guard. This will block most all pieces of glass should a lamp break. It reduces the light and heat emission somewhat, but not significantly. I strongly recommend adding metal window screen to the guard if lamps are overhead and the bather underneath.

Dimmer Switches

Several people have asked about installing dimmer switches on lamps to reduce the intensity of the rays. This could be done. However, dimmers emit strong electromagnetic fields that extend some distance away from the dimmer. For this reason, I do not recommend using dimmer switches.

To reduce the intensity of the lamps, one can place a piece of metal window screen in front of the lamps as part of the lamp guard. One can also move further away from the lamps or even unscrew one lamp to reduce the intensity of the rays. If one decides to use a dimmer switch, be sure it can handle the wattage of the lamps.

Looking At Reddish Infrared Lamps

Many people ask if it is safe to look at the infrared lamps. According to Sylvania Company, the lamps are safe to look at. Indeed, near infrared may have beneficial effects on the retina (*Proc Natl Acad Sci*, 2003, March 7).

The lamps produce very little if any UV-C at all. UV-C is the ultraviolet frequency range found in sunlight that is associated with the development of cataracts and skin cancer.

A few people are sensitive to the light. I suggest using sunglasses if this occurs. Another solution is to add a 75-100-watt full-spectrum bulb to your sauna such as GE Reveal or Chromalux. This may have the added advantage of producing some vitamin D as well. I do not recommend staring at the lamps, but keeping the eyes open appears to be safe and may be helpful for some conditions. I estimate about two to three thousand people are using infrared lamp saunas at the time of this printing (2006). I have had no reports so far that anyone's vision has been harmed by the lamps.

Rotating The Body During A Sauna Session

If one begins to feel a burning sensation in an infrared lamp sauna, it is time to rotate. By wiping off the sweat one may reduce the sensation and may be able to maintain one's position for another minute or two.

On some days the body may be more sensitive to the heat than on others. Perhaps this is due to muscle tension, fatigue or other factors. Also, one area of the body may accept more of the radiant energy than another and this may vary from day to day. Relaxing, breathing deeply and visualizing the body accepting the energy may increase the time a part of the body can tolerate exposure to the heat lamps.

Other Lamp Sauna Considerations

Among the many reports I have received, most everyone is satisfied and reports excellent results with their infrared lamp sauna. However, I have sought negative reports and received a few. Several had enough difficulty to discontinue sauna use.

One person developed a serious ear infection soon after starting sauna therapy. She had a history of ear infections and this was most likely a retracing reaction. However, it affected her balance and she had to discontinue sauna use for about a month. Then she was able to resume and has been well ever since.

Another patient developed a fever and night sweats within several days of beginning sauna therapy. He had a history of pneumonia. He persisted with the saunas for several weeks, as usually these flare-ups go away. His fever persisted and he decided to discontinue its use.

A third patient with an undiagnosed pain syndrome experienced increased pain in the body soon after beginning saunas. He stopped the saunas and the pain subsided. This, too, was probably a healing reaction, but frightened the person sufficiently to cause him to cease using saunas. This, unfortunately, happens frequently.

A fourth patient developed fever and night sweats and had to stop sauna therapy. He had elevated hair mercury and an exhaustion pattern on the hair analysis. All these patients had very low sodium/potassium ratios on their hair mineral analyses, indicating lowered vitality. It is important to note that many others with the same imbalances, however, have had no difficulties other than usual temporary healing reactions after several months to over a year of infrared lamp sauna therapy.

The three most important issues I have encountered with infrared lamp sauna therapy are:

- Some people are reluctant to purchase or build a lamp sauna unit. They object to the cost or the nature of the therapy.
- Some begin a sauna program spending more than about 40 minutes at one time in a sauna. This may cause healing reactions because some people are not acclimated to saunas and sweating may be insufficient. These reactions are upsetting, though not dangerous in our experience. It is always best to begin with no more than 20-30 minutes in a sauna until the body acclimates to sweating and the skin and other organs of elimination begin to function better.

  Those with a four-low-electrolytes pattern on a hair mineral analysis in which the hair has not been washed at the laboratory appear to have the most difficulty. This is not surprising, as this pattern is associated with fatigue, allergies and exhaustion at times. To learn more about this mineral analysis pattern, see Appendix A.
- Even when people begin slowly, healing reactions occasionally occur that frighten people and cause them to abandon the sauna therapy program.

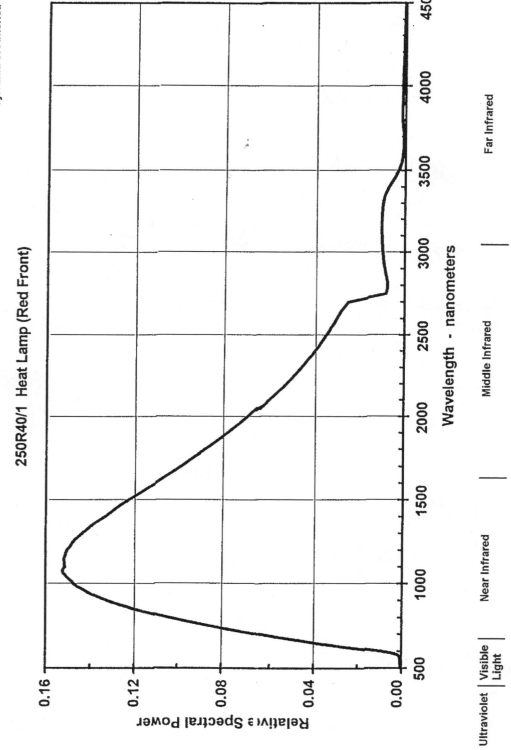

250R40/1 Heat Lamp (Red Front)

Data Courtesy of Osram Sylvania
Sylvania of America- 2003

115

116

14
Personal Experience With An Infrared Lamp Sauna

This chapter is my personal story of using an infrared lamp sauna for therapy. It is included in the book as it may be useful for others.

Sauna Protocol

For a year, I used an infrared lamp sauna upon awakening and just before bed. For the first few months, sessions were limited to 30 minutes. After a few months, the sessions were longer, often 45-50 minutes each. After about eight months, three times I stayed in for 90 minutes at a time. I opened the door about 1/4" when the temperature reached 110-115° F. This prevented the sauna from getting hotter and made the experience much more comfortable. I do not believe a higher temperature is required in an infrared lamp sauna. I had converted a small traditional sauna by adding four lamps to it in a diamond-shaped pattern. I later disconnected the lamp at the feet as I felt it unnecessary and too easy to accidentally hit with my feet.

I drank four ounces of water before entering the sauna and at least eight ounces afterwards. I entered the sauna when it was cold to obtain maximum exposure to the rays. Occasionally I preheated it for 10 minutes or so before entering. Light sweating usually began in about five minutes and the amount of sweat and the areas of the body that sweated most varied greatly over the months. At first sweating remained light, especially certain areas such as the head. The amount of sweating increased several fold as the months went by.

Every few minutes or so the heat caused me to rotate 90° to avoid a slight burn. My skin usually reddened in places for up to an hour after a session and then returned to normal. Sweating became more profuse when the temperature reached about 100° F. Over the months, the experience became more pleasant. At first, I felt exhausted after each session and had to rest afterwards 15 minutes or more. Later, it was less tiring and 10 minutes rest afterward was usually sufficient. Resting after sauna sessions is very important for maximum detoxification.

During the therapy, strenuous exercise or anything else that would deplete energy was minimized, so as to conserve energy for sauna therapy. I lost 12 pounds within about six months. This was a lot, as I was quite thin to begin with. I slowly gained it back over the next six months. Even thin people will lose poor quality tissue on a detoxification program. I made no effort to either gain or lose weight. Saunas can be helpful, however, as part of a weight loss program if one is overweight. This topic is discussed in more detail in Chapter 2.

Healing Reactions

The variety and intensity of healing reactions with the sauna therapy were impressive. For 25 years I have worked on my health as I returned from medical school in Mexico exhausted and depleted. I had experienced many healing reactions before with other natural therapies, so I was surprised that quite a few more occurred with the use of the infrared sauna.

I mention this so others can be prepared for similar reactions. The intensity may have been enhanced by a careful diet, plenty of rest and avoiding all unnecessary stress. For example, I did not travel except for one overnight vacation by car during the entire program, and there I used the sauna at the hotel.

I had excellent supervision and support. This is important as anyone can become concerned when vigorous healing reactions occur. Perception may become altered during a reaction, making one confused or frightened. Though I have plenty of experience with healing reactions, several times I needed to call someone for feedback as to what was occurring and how to proceed.

Fatigue. Though I considered myself healthy, soon after starting sauna therapy I experienced periods of extreme fatigue. At any time of the day, I would suddenly have to lie down and rest for half an hour. At times this was accompanied by a toxic, sick feeling. Usually the fatigue and toxic feeling would pass in less than an hour. At times, a chiropractor had to do energy work to rebalance the body so that energy would return. Rest periods for 15 to 60 minutes at a time were also very important.

The energy level slowly stabilized after eight months, and by the end of the year my energy level was definitely better and more consistent than when I began. I also needed about two hours less sleep per night than when I began.

Aches and Pains. A muscle pain began in the left shoulder, moved down the arm into the hand and then slowly faded over a period of two months. A ligament in the left hand became painful for several months and then cleared up. At one point, the cranial bones shifted, causing the shape of my head to change slightly. This was most unusual and accompanied by a severe headache for a few days. Once, a severe headache lasted five days. Chiropractic and foot reflexology were helpful for headaches. Leg cramps occurred and lasted about three months.

I experienced pains in the kidneys, ureters and testicles. These usually lasted no more than an hour. I drank extra water and rested more when these occurred. At times I experienced sudden sharp pains in the jaws, teeth and gums. They would go away as suddenly as they began. At times the teeth felt loose and then were fine. After a few months, I noticed that a space that had always existed between my front teeth had closed up. Some of the jaw pain I believe was an old cavitation that was slowly cleaned out. Several other patients experienced flare-ups of tooth and gum infections. They were painful, but resolved without complications in a few days to a week. Some symptoms may have been eliminations of Novocain from previous dental procedures.

Bowel symptoms. A number of times I needed to have a bowel movement in the middle of a sauna session. For a month, I was constipated. Four to seven tablets of GB-3 (ox bile and pancreatin) per meal were needed to have one movement per day.

Later I had diarrhea for a week. Each time I stepped into the sauna, in five minutes or so I heard gurgling in the gall bladder area and had to run to the bathroom. This may have been a toxin that irritated the intestines. I also believe I eliminated stored antibiotics, of which I had taken a lot as a child. As these were eliminated in the bile, they may have destroyed the intestinal flora. I began taking large doses of acidophilus and the diarrhea cleared up.

Gas pains occasionally occurred suddenly that were quite severe. Pain would sometimes radiate up to the chest. I would lie down and they would pass in fifteen minutes to an hour. These gas attacks gradually subsided as the months went on.

Skin Rashes. When I began the program, I had itchy eczema on both hands that had persisted several years and resisted all treatment. It cleared up completely after 10 months of sauna therapy. My heels became very dry and crusted after a few months on the sauna program. This slowly went away and the heels became soft and supple. The skin on my hands and fingers had been very dry with occasional cracking in our cold, dry winters. After sauna therapy for a year, the skin was and still is much softer and more moist.

Most people experience some type of skin eliminations and rashes that can occur on any part of the body. The legs or abdomen are common sites. These generally fade away after several days to weeks.

Infections. I retraced a sinus condition for three days with a mild fever and a headache. Asthmatic retracing then began. I had had asthma as a child, but with no symptoms for 30 years. Asthma symptoms ended with bronchitis that lasted two days. Perhaps this was how it began at age two or three.

Several weeks later I retraced hepatitis from twenty-five years before. My liver ached, I was tired and slightly feverish. This lasted several weeks. I took bee propolis and other supplements for viral infections. I also retraced other infections that caused flu-like symptoms for a day or two.

Later, I retraced an eye infection I had had years before. Pain flared up for about an hour and then subsided. Later, it flared up two more times. I also experienced night sweats for several weeks. These may have been due to an old tubercular infection or pneumonia that flared up as it healed.

Odors. One evening I coughed up a foul-tasting secretion. Several times foul odors occurred in the sauna including that of pesticides, rotten eggs and rotten fish. These usually passed in a few minutes. The rotten egg odor was perhaps due to sulfur compounds that bind and help transport copper. The rotten fish odor may have been due to proteins that bind mercury as it is eliminated. Protein binding is important to minimize the toxicity of these metals as they are being eliminated. On several occasions, a chlorine odor filled the sauna. I used to swim often in chlorinated pools.

Emotional Reactions. These usually took the form of strange, violent or fearful dreams, or feelings of anxiety. Some anxiety I attribute to eliminating caffeine or toxic metals such as copper.

Computer Sensitivity. A very welcome change I attribute to sauna therapy was a reduction in sensitivity to newer computers. For several years I had had to avoid new computers, as they caused severe headaches. It may have been due to an ultrasound frequency as it was less if I used earplugs. The type of monitor did not matter. I had to use an old Pentium 90 machine that did not cause the problem. After nine months of sauna therapy, the headaches began to improve and I can now tolerate the newer machines, particularly an Apple I-Book laptop.

Validation

During sauna therapy, I did a hair mineral analysis every two to three months. These are included at the end of this section. Some of the changes during sauna therapy are summarized in the two charts below.

To read these charts, the numbers (1 through 7) along the bottom of the graphs indicate sequential hair analysis retests. The numbers along the left side indicate the mineral levels in milligrams per 100 grams. To obtain levels in parts per million, multiply these numbers by 10.

The charts show dramatic increases in iron, aluminum, manganese and chromium during sauna therapy. *When a mineral level rises rapidly on a retest hair mineral analysis, in almost every case it indicates a significant elimination of that mineral.*

Such great increases in mineral levels at a time when I was very careful as to what I ate, drank, breathed or touched, indicates an elimination of these metals through the skin and hair. After an initial increase, on each successive test, the numbers declined back toward normal, indicating a reduced rate of elimination as the sauna program progressed.

The numbers are quite dramatic by any standards. In twenty-five years of testing my mineral levels during many natural therapy programs, I had never had readings anywhere near these levels. In fact, I had never shown high levels of iron, manganese or chromium though I had seen them in many others. The dramatic elevations, especially on the first test performed after about a month of sauna therapy, showed me that indeed infrared lamp sauna therapy is most helpful for removing toxic levels of metals. No other therapy I have experienced has shown this ability to such an extent.

Hair Mineral Values For One Year During Sauna Therapy

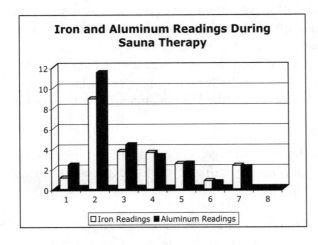

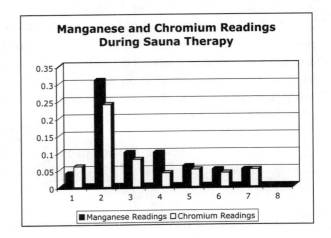

I was surprised to see the metal eliminations, although they help explain the healing reactions. I had lived in Mexico for five years, have had some pesticide exposure and grew up eating my share of junk food. I have found that most people have excess amounts of iron, manganese and aluminum in particular. Often they will not be eliminated except through the use of the sauna.

Iron, manganese and chromium are essential minerals. However, if unable to be used correctly, or in certain forms, these essential minerals become toxic. Iron becomes toxic if copper is not available to change it from the ferric to the ferrous form. Chromium and manganese can oxidize, and become toxic in this form. They can contribute to liver, kidney, heart and brain disorders. Iron, manganese, chromium and aluminum can help maintain the sodium level and act as compensatory mechanisms in adrenal exhaustion. I had had adrenal exhaustion at one time. Sources of manganese include gasoline. Iron comes from refined flour products, cookware, vitamin pills and other sources. Chromium and aluminum are other common environmental contaminants.

Aluminum has no known physiological role. It accumulates in the kidneys and brain where it can affect memory and cognition. I had been very careful for many years to avoid sources of aluminum such as table salt, antacids, anti-perspirants, aluminum cookware and beverages in aluminum cans.

After nine months, the manganese and aluminum levels were still elevated. Even with two saunas daily and a very relaxed and healthful lifestyle, correction was slow. This is why a three-week or three-month detoxification program is not enough for many people.

Lead began to rise on the later tests. It represents a deeper layer of toxins. Most people have layers and layers of toxins. We are born with some of them. Exposures from food, water, air and contact with toxic substances just add to the burden. They cause many illnesses, both physical and mental.

The calcium and magnesium levels increased after two months of sauna therapy and remained elevated for months. I took only a minimal amount of calcium and magnesium supplements, although I ate a lot of kelp during the first four months of the program. I believe the elevation was an elimination through the hair of stored, biounavailable calcium and magnesium. Later, arsenic increased as deeper layers of toxins were eliminated.

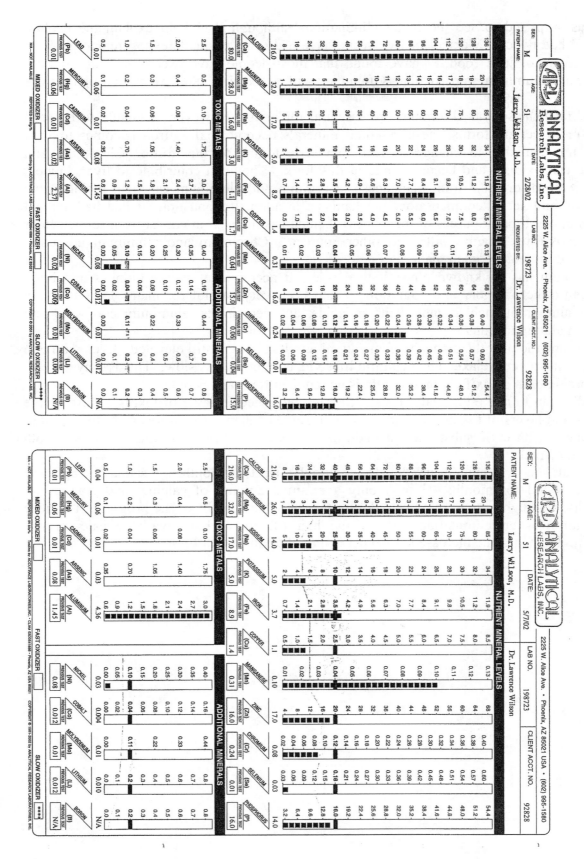

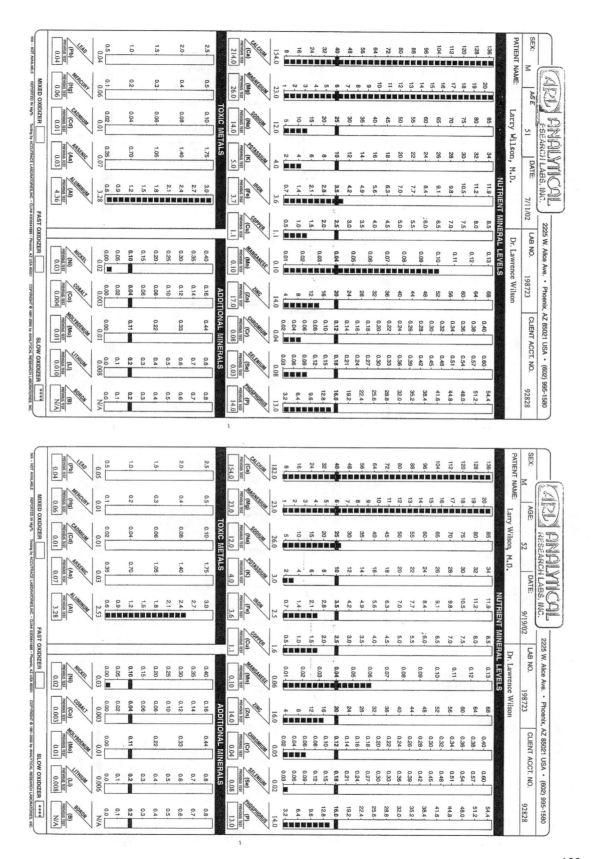

123

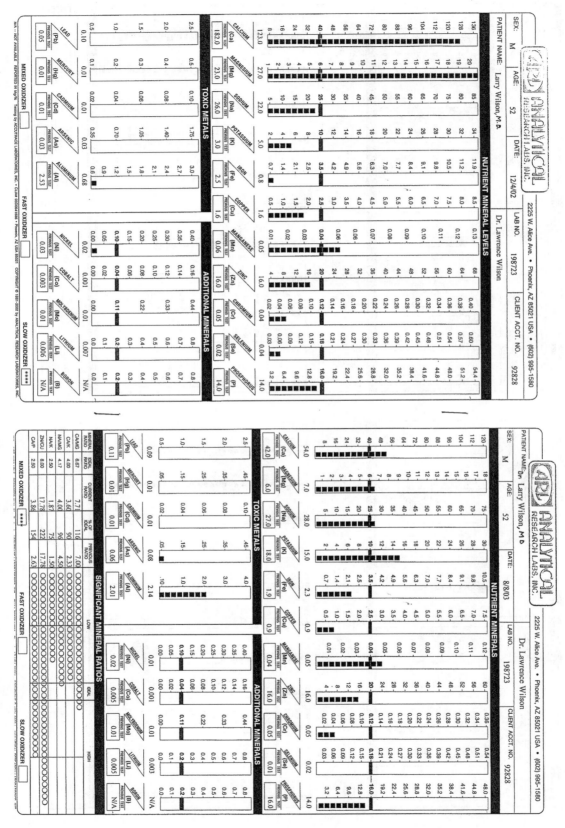

15
Sauna Research

"*Two years ago I was diagnosed with cardiomyopathy and an asthmatic condition, causing a constant cough. I began using an infrared lamp sauna and have used it almost every day for 22 months. The cough has cleared and my heart has gone from "markedly dilated" to "mildly dilated". I have more energy and my thinking is clearer. My cardiologist is very surprised*". - Mr. J.M., Manchester, Connecticut

This book is essentially a research report based on clinical experience and the existing medical literature. I hope it will inspire others to research more deeply into this excellent healing modality. The following suggestions are to assist in designing studies that can shed more light on the mechanisms and physiology involved in sauna therapy.

Research Protocols

Much of the medical literature related to sauna therapy lacks complete details. Setting up research studies properly is important to avoid confusion and conflicting results. Addressing the research concerns below would greatly assist in developing a more exact science of sauna therapy.

- Researchers need to state the type of sauna used, the duration and frequency of sessions and the length of the program.

- The metabolic type or oxidation rate of the research subject, in my experience, often causes differing responses to sauna therapy. It would be helpful if researchers would use hair mineral analysis or other standardized methods to assess body chemistry, rather than simply classifying subjects by their age, gender, symptoms or health conditions.

- The research subjects' diet, amount of rest and activity level are extremely important. For example, vigorous exercise or inadequate rest result in more sympathetic nervous system activity. This can greatly reduce the effectiveness of sauna detoxification. One's diet may enhance energy or use it up, with significant effects on sauna therapy outcomes.

- The research subjects' total body load of important toxins may affect the outcome of a program. Toxic exposures include past and present use of synthetic drugs, both prescription and recreational. It is also helpful to know of other toxic exposures to solvents, metals, radiation, dental amalgams and other toxic agents. Some herbal formulas and minerals from earth or sea deposits are high in toxic metals, especially if used daily.

- Sauna researchers need to clearly distinguish between effects that occur *during a single sauna session* and *long-term effects* resulting from repeated sauna use in a therapy program. For example, the heart rate may increase during a single sauna session. However, repeated sauna use may lead to a reduced resting heart rate. The same may occur with other measurements such as hormones and blood sugar levels.

- Narrative descriptions of clinical experiences are important, perhaps more so than reporting 'average' results. Some effects of sauna therapy are similar for everyone, such as reduced liver and kidney toxicity. However, experiences during sauna detoxification programs may vary greatly with each individual. Also, the time required for detoxification may vary significantly, even among those of the same age, gender, occupation or health condition. Each has been exposed to different toxins over a lifetime. Stress levels vary a lot. Also, some were also born more toxic or with weaker organs or glands.

- Researchers need to be able to distinguish physiological effects of sauna use from temporary healing reactions. For example, the release of stored caffeine during sauna sessions may cause irritability. From this, it would be incorrect to conclude that sauna therapy always causes irritability.

Research Topics

Research is needed as to the most effective type of sauna for detoxification, particular toxins that can or cannot be eliminated through sauna therapy and the best sauna protocols for various conditions such as acute infections, chronic illnesses and others.

In addition, more safety studies are needed, especially on the newer far infrared and infrared lamp saunas. I have found, for example, that after several years of intense use of an infrared lamp sauna, less exposure to the lamps appears better.

Sauna Therapy Program Features

For the best evaluation of sauna therapy, here are some guidelines for setting up research protocols:

- **The therapy program should be undertaken for specifically described reasons or conditions**. These may include drug addiction, illness, emotional release or eliminating metals or chemicals. One should be able to measure achievement of the goal.

126

- **A thorough program involves spending from 30 minutes up to one or even more hours in a sauna several times a week or preferably daily. The program or trial needs to last for several weeks to a year or more.**

- **Other modalities should ideally be combined with sauna therapy.** Adjuncts may include visualization, color or sound in the sauna. Additional therapies may include vitamin and mineral supplements, herbs, diets, massage and other therapies. Studies using only the sauna definitely have merit. However, the results will be best when sauna therapy is part of a more complete healing program.

- **The program should be supervised, at least by phone, by someone with experience with sauna therapy and natural healing programs.** Sauna therapy is not strictly a do-it-yourself therapy, although it may be done at home. Supervision and moral support are helpful for everyone. Otherwise, when healing reactions occur, it is easy to become discouraged or frightened and stop the program. Healing or purification reactions can affect one's judgment. Input from another knowledgeable person at these times is most helpful.

- **The program needs to be structured, yet also flexible.** Each person and each condition are somewhat different. Also, the protocol may need to be modified at times to respond to changes that occur day to day.

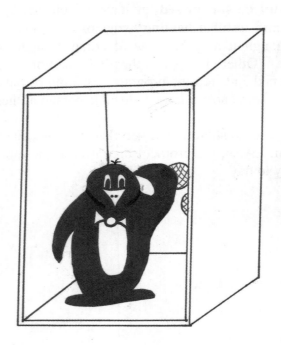

*"Even I can stand to be
in this infrared lamp sauna."*

16
Review and Conclusion

"I suffered from fatigue, food allergies and other digestive difficulties. I experienced swollen lymph nodes as well. I began using an infrared lamp sauna every day, eight months ago, and am delighted with the results. The sauna boosts my energy, the swollen lymph nodes have gone away and I feel much healthier." - Mrs. S.K., Nashville, TN

Hot air baths have been used for thousands of years for recreation, health maintenance, social gathering and spiritual renewal. Their value as a therapeutic method is common knowledge, empirically demonstrated and used in many indigenous cultures.

Saunas have been used for many purposes in these cultures and the same, I believe, will happen someday in our own. They are a place of retreat and repose, a place to work out problems and dilemmas, and a place of therapy and healing.

Toxic Metals And Toxic Chemicals

Today, the challenges of toxic metals, harmful chemicals, ionizing radiation and drug-resistant pathogenic microorganisms make sauna therapy very attractive and even essential for physical healing.

Sauna use inhibits the sympathetic nervous system, dilates peripheral blood vessels and causes profuse sweating. It greatly enhances the circulation of the blood and lymph, increases oxygenation of the tissues and relieves internal organ congestion. It can also help relieve pain, relax muscles and increase the flexibility of tendons and ligaments. It also helps the body kill or disable many microorganisms and hastens the death of weaker, toxic and mutated cells. Producing heat shock proteins may be another great benefit of sauna use.

Infrared

Much of this book is devoted to a look at the power of near infrared energy. It is a most fascinating subject for scientific investigation. Near infrared energy produced by the reddish heat lamps will be found, I believe, to be a primary tissue nutrient that can increase oxygen production, reduce lipid peroxidation, and decouple toxins from water molecules. If continued research bears out this assertion, it would make sense that every household should have a near infrared lamp sauna in the home as a basic piece of furniture similar to a bathtub or a stove.

Saunas And Detoxification

Saunas are best known for their ability and their use to assist detoxification. This critical body function is impaired in almost everyone today. Saunas can move toxic metals, toxic chemicals and other types of biological toxins out of the body, often in ways few other therapies can match at any cost.

Chronic Infections

Saunas are also helpful to resolve chronic infections of many types. I believe that research will demonstrate the immense value of saunas for infectious diseases, perhaps surpassing their value for detoxification and other purposes. Every home could use an infrared lamp sauna today as insurance and rapid treatment for infectious conditions.

Other Health Conditions

Experience and a growing amount of research also demonstrate the benefits of sauna therapy for many other health conditions including cancer and heart disease, among others. These benefits are so great that I hope they will be recognized by the established medical community in time to save many lives while sparing the pocketbook as well. I have no doubt that sauna therapy will take its place one day as a premier treatment modality for these and so many other pressing health concerns in our world.

Spiritual Renewal

A number of clients report that they use their sauna as a sanctuary and place of worship. Some keep rosary beads in the sauna. Others report that they write prayers on pieces of paper and tack them to the walls of the sauna. Some also set up a music system to provide peaceful and religious music. In the Native American tradition, and perhaps others, the sauna is considered a place of renewal of the body, mind and spirit, and a place of retreat and healing.

Other Modalities Combined

Color therapy provided by infrared lamps enhances the activity of the eliminative organs and appears to affect the emotional body as well. The sauna is also an excellent place to employ conscious breathing, reflexology, sound therapy, visualization, and perhaps other modalities as well. When thus combined into a total health program, the sauna becomes even more effective and powerful as a holistic healing therapy.

Conclusion

Sauna therapy is beginning to take its place as a primary healing modality. More research, study and experimentation are much needed to confirm or disprove the observations presented in this text. I look forward to the day when sauna use will be a regular part of our lifestyles, as common as television sets and used just as often.

We will use saunas before having children to give them the best start in life possible. We will continue to use the gentle heat of the sauna for prevention of illness, protection against environmental chemicals and metals, and to treat our own and our families' ailments. The need for this simple, powerful method of detoxification and healing has never been greater.

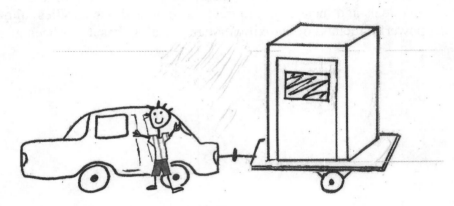

"Okay, honey, I'm ready to leave for vacation"

APPENDICES

Appendix A. Saunas And Hair Mineral Analysis

This appendix brings together insights from mineral analysis research as they apply to sauna therapy. I have specialized in the use of hair tissue mineral testing for 34 years. I have written a large textbook about it entitled *Nutritional Balancing and Hair Mineral Analysis*. Even more information about hair mineral testing is found at www.drlwilson.com.

Hair mineral analysis can be useful to assess a person's tendency for toxicity, their detoxification ability and their overall vitality or energy level. It can also identify electrolyte imbalances that could make sauna use somewhat more hazardous.

Hair mineral analysis can also be used to monitor progress to some degree on a sauna therapy program. One can easily and with little cost observe toxic metal eliminations, changes in metabolism called the oxidation rate and watch other mineral patterns shift during the program. To a degree, a properly performed and interpreted hair mineral analysis can also guide dietary and supplement recommendations that can enhance a sauna therapy program.

Procedural Matters. In our experience, *hair **must not be washed** at the laboratory for accurate electrolyte readings*. This is an important aspect of hair analysis interpretation. See the web site, www.drlwilson.com for an in-depth discussion of this topic.

To understand and interpret a hair analysis correctly, I strongly suggest the method of interpretation devised by the late Dr. Paul C. Eck. This is also explained more fully on my web site.

All mineral values in this appendix are reported in milligrams per hundred grams (mg%). To convert to parts per million (ppm), as reported by some laboratories, multiply the readings by 10. Mineral ratios do not need converting.

The Tendency For Toxicity

Slow Oxidation. When a hair sodium/magnesium ratio is less than 4.17:1 and the hair calcium/potassium ratio is greater than 4:1, Dr. Paul Eck called the pattern *slow oxidation*. Note that the term slow oxidation is used somewhat differently by other researchers. The hair must not be washed at the laboratory for accurate readings.

About ninety percent of adults are in this group. These individuals are often cold, often do not sweat easily, and tend to be more toxic than fast oxidizers. Their thyroid and adrenal glands tend to be underactive.

They do best with daily or twice daily sauna sessions. They also benefit greatly from longer sauna sessions, although everyone should begin with 20-minute sessions for the first few days to weeks until their bodies acclimate to sweating.

Fast Oxidation. Dr. Eck defined *fast oxidation* as the condition when the hair sodium/magnesium ratio is greater than 4.17:1 and the hair calcium/potassium ratio is less than 4:1. Once again, the hair must not be washed at the laboratory for accurate readings.

Fast oxidizers with a sodium/potassium ratio of 2.5 or greater and a calcium level of 40 mg% or less are called *true fast oxidizers*. These individuals tend to sweat more easily and often have a slightly higher body temperature due to greater adrenal and thyroid glandular activity. Some of them are slightly less toxic because they are more able to eliminate toxins. However, this is not always the case, especially if their hair mineral test reveals *poor eliminator patterns*.

Healthy fast oxidizers, who are rare, may require somewhat less time in a sauna or less frequent sauna sessions. They may also be more heat-sensitive. They should begin with only about three sessions per week, and work up to once a day. If the magnesium level is 2 mg% or less, or if the calcium level is 14 mg% or less, be sure to begin with only 20 minutes per session. They must drink plenty of spring water before and after a sauna session.

Many who appear as fast oxidizers will change within a few months to slow oxidation. Their fast oxidation pattern was, in fact, only due to temporary stress. Others will alternate between fast and slow oxidation. Young children are often fast oxidizers. This is one reason to exercise more care with children in saunas.

Four Low Electrolytes. A hair calcium level less than 40 mg%, magnesium less than 6 mg%, sodium less than 25 mg% and potassium less than 10 mg% is a pattern called *four low electrolytes*. It is associated with exhaustion, often allergies, chronic stress and eventually debility. These individuals are often very toxic. However, this is often not revealed on the hair mineral analysis because of their impaired ability to eliminate toxins. Their sympathetic nervous systems are chronically stimulated, reducing their ability to detoxify. These people may have more difficulty with sauna therapy. Begin with 15-20 minutes in a sauna and limit sessions to four per week, at least for the first month, to be on the safe side.

A Low Sodium/Potassium Ratio or Inversion. When a hair sodium/potassium ratio is less than 2.5:1, the pattern is called a *sodium/potassium inversion*. When the ratio is less than 1:1, the pattern is considered severe or a *trauma Na/K ratio*. It is associated with exhaustion, carbohydrate intolerance, chronic stress, a tendency for chronic infections and often debility. Toxicity is generally greater in these individuals. Begin with 20-minute sessions and a maximum of five sessions per week. The hair must not be washed at the laboratory in order to obtain accurate sodium and potassium readings.

Detoxification Ability

The list below is a rough guide as to which metabolic types detoxify most easily. Those who detoxify most easily are listed first. There can be exceptions depending on environmental or other factors.

- True fast oxidizers (those with a Ca/K less than 4, Na/Mg greater than 4.17, Na/K greater than 2.5:1, Ca less than 40 mg% and Mg less than 6 mg%).
- Fast oxidizers with a Na/K ratio less than 2.0.
- Mild slow oxidizers (those with a Ca/K greater than 4, Na/Mg less than 4.17, Na/K greater than 2:1 and a Ca/K ratio less than about 20:1).
- Moderate slow oxidizers (those with a Na/K ratio less than 2:1 and greater than 1:1 or a Ca/K ratio greater than 20 and less than 100).

- Extreme slow oxidizers (those with a Ca/K greater than 100:1 or a Na/K ratio between 1:1 and 2:1).
- Four low electrolytes or a slow oxidizer with a sodium/potassium ratio less than 1.0.

More Hazardous Electrolyte Imbalances

Limit the length of sauna sessions and/or have more supervision when the following mineral imbalances are present:

1. Extremely low electrolyte levels:
Calcium less than 11 mg%
Magnesium less than 4 mg%
Sodium less than 5 mg%
Potassium less than 3 mg%

2. Extreme Vital Mineral Ratios:
Sodium/potassium ratio less than 1
Calcium/magnesium ratio greater than 15

3. Extreme Fast or Slow Oxidation:
Calcium/potassium ratio less than 0.5
Calcium/potassium ratio greater than 100

The Energy Level

If a person has a very low energy level, it may be wise to begin with less time in a sauna. Hair analysis indicators for low energy include a sodium/potassium ratio less than 1:1, a calcium/potassium ratio greater than 100:1, cadmium greater than 0.02, copper greater than 2.5 or a four low electrolyte pattern (calcium less than 40, magnesium less than 6, sodium less than 25 and potassium less than 10 mg%). Cancer patients are an exception in that they always require two or more sauna sessions daily. Always have excellent supervision if one has a chronic illness, however, such as cancer.

Sympathetic Dominance

A hair potassium level of 4 mg% or less indicates *sympathetic dominance*. This means the person tends to overuse their sympathetic or fight-or-flight nervous system. It is mainly a personality trait, although toxic conditions can play a significant role as well.

Their sympathetic nervous system, including the adrenal glands and thyroid, are generally exhausted, but their mental tendency to fight or run remains. This leads to illness as the sympathetic system is catabolic. Parasympathetic activity is required to nourish, regenerate and eliminate toxins from the body.

Repeated sauna use can be most helpful to help relax these individuals and shift them into a parasympathetic or relaxed state. Many, however, report feeling tired after a sauna session because the sauna tends to shut down the sympathetic nervous system for a time. Autonomic *dominance* is different than one's autonomic *state*. See Appendix B for more information about the autonomic nervous system.

Toxic Metal Readings on Mineral Analyses

Do not be misled by high toxic metal readings on fast oxidizers' mineral tests. These individuals have a greater ability to excrete toxic metals. Thus hair, urine or other readings of these metals may be higher. Those with a more sluggish metabolism, although toxic, cannot excrete as well. Their toxic metals are locked deep within body tissues and are often not revealed at first on hair mineral analyses. Several months or more of sauna use and other therapies may be required before toxic metals are revealed on their mineral analyses.

Another tipoff that a person is more toxic is the presence of *poor eliminator patterns* on a hair mineral analysis. These are extremely low toxic metal levels, and indicate difficulty eliminating toxic metals. Sauna sessions are very important to help resolve this pattern. Please read *Poor Eliminator Pattern* at www.drlwilson.com for more details and criteria for the poor eliminator pattern. It is one of the most important patterns seen on hair mineral tests.

Which Hair Testing Laboratory to Use

Most hair mineral laboratories wash the hair with detergents, alcohol, acetone and other solvents. Hair is 10-15% porous. Chemical washing at the laboratory erratically removes water-soluble elements, especially sodium and potassium.

Most major laboratories are excellent for testing toxic metals in the hair. However, for accurate readings of the water-soluble trace elements, use a lab that does not wash the hair. The water-soluble elements are needed to assess the oxidation rate and for other critical aspects of interpretation as well.

Only two labs, Analytical Research Labs (ARL) and Trace Elements, Inc. do not wash the hair. I recommend ARL for their superior testing and program recommendations. They can be reached at 1-800-528-4067 or www.arltma.com.

At this time (2014), I modify their computer-generated programs for greater effectiveness. I also assist physicians and nutrition consultants to learn how to interpret the tests properly. Anyone interested may contact me at larry@drlwilson.com or (928) 445-7690.

Monitoring Progress

Retesting hair mineral levels every few months can be an excellent way to monitor progress during a sauna therapy program. However, anyone interested in doing this must learn how to intepret the repeated hair mineral analyses correctly. Otherwise, one can be easily misled. I find blood and urine tests less useful to monitor progress.

Appendix B. Restoring The Sympathetic Nervous System

The human nervous system has two major divisions, the *voluntary* and the *autonomic* systems. The *voluntary nervous system* is concerned mainly with cognition, movement and sensation. It consists of motor and sensory nerves, among many others. The *autonomic system* mainly controls functions over which we have less conscious control. These include the digestion of food, the blood pressure and the heart rate. Its nerves leave the spine and connect to all the major organs and glands, either inhibiting or stimulating their activity.

The autonomic system has two branches. These are called the *sympathetic* and the *parasympathetic branches*. Most people who are not well have exhausted their sympathetic system. Restoring balance to the autonomic nervous system is a great secret for healing all health conditions.

The Sympathetic Branch

* The sympathetic branch of the autonomic nervous system activates the glands and organs that defend the body against attack. It is called the fight-or-flight system. Its nerves direct more blood to the muscles and the brain. It causes the heart rate and blood pressure to increase, while blood flow to the digestive and eliminative organs decreases.

It also activates the thyroid and adrenal glands to provide extra energy for fighting or running away. One may feel nervous, irritable or even panicky when in a sympathetic state of readiness.

The sympathetic system is catabolic, which means it tears down the body. Energy is used to prepare for defense, rather than for nourishment or for elimination of wastes. An excellent analogy is to imagine placing all of the nation's resources in its military defense. While helpful in an emergency, if continued too long, the nation becomes much poorer for lack of productive commercial activity. The feeling of an 'adrenalin rush' is a product of the sympathetic system. It may feel good at first, but is always followed by a feeling of fatigue, as this system uses up energy and depletes the body.

The Parasympathetic Branch

* The parasympathetic system of nerves is concerned with nourishing, healing and regeneration of the body. It is *anabolic*, or concerned with rebuilding the body. Its nerves stimulate digestion, and the immune and eliminative organs. These organs include the liver, kidneys, pancreas, stomach and intestines. The parasympathetic nervous system, when activated by rest, relaxation and happy thoughts, is essential for balanced living and for all healing. Moving yourself into a healthy parasympathetic state, and staying there as much of the time as possible, helps heal all health conditions, both physical and emotional ones as well.

The feeling often associated with the parasympathetic state can be one of lethargy or fatigue, as you are so relaxed. Do not, however, believe this is unhealthy. Rather, it indicates a state of repair and rebuilding in progress.

The sympathetic and parasympathetic systems are antagonistic. Either one or the other is activated most all of the time. The sympathetic system, however, always takes precedence, because it is concerned with one's survival.

The sympathetic nervous system may be *roughly* likened to the gas pedal of a car. The parasympathetic is more like the brake. Unlike a car, however, when the 'brake' is applied to the body, it begins to heal itself.

AUTONOMIC IMBALANCES

Let us now examine a balanced autonomic system, and the sympathetic and parasympathetic dominant imbalances.

The Balanced Individual. When the sympathetic and parasympathetic systems are working as they should, the tendency is to rest often and easily. One can, however, perform at "top speed" with equal ease. When challenged by stress, the balanced person is able to respond with vigor and fortitude.

The parasympathetic system reduces the activity of the brain, the muscles, and the adrenal and thyroid glands. When no situation is pressing, the balanced person can comfortably choose to rest and can sleep deeply.

Sympathetic Dominance. Most people today overuse their sympathetic nervous system. They do not spend enough time in a parasympathetic state to fully rebuild their bodies. Their bodies eventually become nutritionally depleted and they become quite literally 'burned out'. Today, even children are often burned out, in this sense, due to stress, poor diets and nutritional deficiencies they are born with. This is revealed on a hair mineral analysis as a slow oxidation rate, and particularly when the hair potassium level is less than about 4 mg% or the sodium/potassium ratio is greater than about 5.

The causes for sympathetic dominance vary. Some people take on too much work. Others analyze too much or worry excessively. Others live in fear, anger or resentment too much of the time. A person in this condition may also talk, think, eat or work at a rapid pace, faster than the optimum for that person. One also becomes more toxic and nutritionally depleted, which sets up a vicious cycle at times that perpetuates the pattern, or at least makes the condition worse.

Once accustomed to sympathetic dominance, a second vicious cycle often occurs. A person can become so used to being tired that if, by chance, he gets a lot of rest one day, the person will often use up their energy the next day, instead of continuing to rest. That is, one does not allow oneself to use the energy they accumulated for healing and rebuilding because the concept and feelings involved in resting and rebuilding have become foreign. As a result of theses two vicious cycles, people tend to stay in sympathetic dominance and remain depleted and out of balance.

The early signs of staying in a sympathetic dominant state too much of the time include fatigue, anxiety at times and perhaps feelings of exhaustion. As the condition progresses, one may feel more anxious, depressed, moody or apathetic. Other physical symptoms include aches and pains, weakness, disturbed digestion and insomnia. If this state of the nervous system continues, the stage is set for more serious illness.

138

Parasympathetic Dominance. This can be of two types, healthy and unhealthy. The healthy state is encountered rarely. It occurs only in what might be called spiritually developed people. They live most of their lives in the present moment. They are almost always relaxed, do not react to stress and live in a state of peace and contentment.

Much more common today is an unhealthy parasympathetic state. It is basically an end stage result of sympathetic dominance. People in this condition have exhausted their sympathetic systems so much, they have flipped into a parasympathetic state by default. They cannot fight back as well as they used to. They are essentially in a state of give-up or hopelessness about their situation or health condition.

The causes of the healthy and unhealthy parasympathetic states are quite opposite. Healthy parasympathetic dominance is due to what may be called personal development. This is the discipline to think and live differently. One reduces stress and strain on the body by resting and nourishing it so that it can rebuild. Meditation and other practices can help to discipline the thoughts and emotions to remain in a balanced state of mind.

Unhealthy parasympathetic dominance, as stated earlier, is quite the opposite. It is the result of overworking the sympathetic nervous system until it no longer functions adequately and one goes into a give-up state. Symptoms may include feeling depressed and cynical. Some are paralyzed by their fear or anger about their situation. This, coupled with nutritional imbalances, sets the stage for serious illness and emotional disorders as well.

Today, fearful thinking, electromagnetic pollution, toxic metals and toxic chemicals in the food, air and water all disturb the functioning of the autonomic system. As a result, healthy autonomic nervous system activity is unusual.

BALANCING THE AUTONOMIC SYSTEM

Sauna therapy is one of the finest ways to gently inhibit the activity of the sympathetic nervous system, which can help allow the system to rebalance and rebuild. In addition, the following lifestyle modifications are also extremely helpful.

- *Rest Often.* Nap often, and sleep at least 8 hours or more each night. The hours before midnight are by far the best for sleeping. Avoid excessive activity of any kind. Even exercise is often overdone. Exercise is a powerful sympathetic stimulant. Avoid getting exhausted by any activity you engage in. Be careful when using exercise to "run away" from stress, for example. More rest is often what is really required.
- *Eat Well.* The nervous system must be properly nourished to function correctly. High quality animal protein is particularly helpful for the brain and nervous system as it contains fats and proteins essential for the nerves. These include the omega-3 and omega-6 essential fatty acids. Excellent foods for the nervous system are eggs, meats, nuts, root vegetables and oily fish such as sardines and salmon. See Chapter 7 for more information about diet.
- *Reduce Excessive And Harmful Stress.* Stress is the main activator of the sympathetic nervous system. Stress can arise from within the body due to fatigue, muscle tension, spinal misalignment or nutritional deficiencies, among other reasons. Other sources of stress are worry, fears, anger, guilt and negative thinking.

Stress can also come from outside, such as financial, work or family stress. Other types of stress to minimize or avoid are living in a noisy environment, or in one with contaminated air and water.

Electromagnetic stress is also very real, although it cannot be seen. Reduce your use of computers if possible, and do not keep televisions, computers and other electrical devices on when not in use. Be sure to turn them all off when you sleep, and keep even clocks and radios away from your head in the location where you sleep. Activities like city driving and using cell phones are also stress-producing, even if you are not aware of it at the time. A simple lifestyle is much preferred.

- *Keep One's Thoughts And Emotions As Uplifted And Positive As Possible, All Of The Time. Train your mind to stay out of negative emotions. These include worry, fear, anger and guilt.* These emotions turn on the sympathetic system and keep it active. Meditation, affirmations, counseling and other natural therapies can all help. Also, surround yourself only with uplifting books, tapes and other forms of media. Pick your friends and relationships carefully. Work, school and all your activities either contribute to your contentment or detract from it.

- *Stay In gratitude.* This will help keep you in a positive, uplifted state. Keeping a gratitude journal can be very helpful. Each evening, write down five things you are grateful for this day.

- *Practice Forgiveness.* This places you in a position of power and compassion. It is much better than allowing yourself to feel like a victim, which always leads to a fight-or-flight response.

- *Cultivate Contentment.* This is different from feeling you need to be happy all the time. Happiness, as most people know it, is often short-lived. It is often an attempt to overcome feelings of unhappiness. Contentment is a state in which you are at peace with yourself and the world, even if the world around you is not to your liking. You can learn to let the world go and choose contentment rather than attempting always to control the world.

- *Do Not Compare Yourself With Others.* This causes fear, and often anger and resentment. The world never seems fair from our limited perspectives. There is much that is hidden. If you knew more about others' lives, you would be less anxious to trade places with them.

- *Breathe Deeply.* This is one way to control the autonomic system with a voluntary action. Slow, deep breathing by itself turns off the sympathetic system.

- *Supplemental Nutrients May Be Most Helpful.* Nutrients that may help relax the sympathetic system include calcium, magnesium, zinc and B-complex vitamins, particularly from foods such as nutritional yeast, meats and eggs. High doses of B-complex vitamins are rarely needed or helpful. Other calming nutrients include GABA, L-taurine and L-carnitine. Herbs that calm the nervous system include valerian, passionflower, skullcap and hops, among others.

CONCLUSION

Understanding the basics of the autonomic nervous system is extremely important for your health and well-being. Overstimulation and eventually exhaustion of the sympathetic system is an enormous problem today that contributes to almost any health condition by impairing nutrition, elimination and immune system activity. Sauna therapy over a period of time is a powerful way to help rebalance the autonomic nervous system.

Appendix C. Notes For Practitioners

Some people will not build or buy a sauna for their home, although I believe that most could use one. Detoxification centers are needed where clients can use saunas for prevention, detoxification, relaxation, health maintenance and as part of natural healing programs. Offering sauna therapy at one's office or clinic is an excellent addition to any practice. Saunas will enhance the effects of most other therapeutic modalities.

The simplicity and low construction and operating costs of an infrared lamp sauna offer practitioners a way to provide this service at rates reasonable enough to allow clients to use the facility several times a week.

Sauna therapy can be offered on a fully supervised basis or the practitioner can set up a sauna program and clients carry it out on their own, checking with the practitioner when needed.

Sauna Disclaimer Statement

Practitioners offering sauna therapy may wish to use a simple disclaimer statement such as the following:

Sauna therapy is a way of enhancing circulation, decongesting internal organs and increasing the activity of the skin through the application of heat to the body. It is not a diagnosis, treatment, prescription or cure for any health condition, nor is it intended to replace regular health care.

Signed_____ Date_____

Appendix D. Infrared Sauna Electrical Unit Plans

The infrared lamp sauna described here performs superbly. Essentially, one builds an electrical unit consisting of three infrared heat lamps mounted on a piece of wood. You can place this unit in a sauna enclosure or in a small bathroom or small closet. The simplest enclosure is a frame covered with fabric. Plans for this enclosure follow the plans for the electrical unit.

Materials

- **Three 250-watt, red, incandescent "heat lamps".** These are sold at many hardware stores. *Do not use clear heat lamps* as their spectrum is not correct. My preferences are *Philips, General Electric, Sylvania, Feit, Halco or Havel-Sli lamps. Westinghouse* lamps are somewhat acceptable. At the time of this printing (2014) Westinghouse may be coating their lamps with Teflon. This reduces the danger of breakage, but the lamps may outgas when hot.

- **Three ceramic or plastic lamp sockets designed for 250-watt bulbs.** Sockets are available that wire from the front or from the back. Another type of socket unscrews so that one places half the socket behind a thin piece of wood or metal.

- **Fifteen feet of heavy lamp cord, a medium duty male wall plug and a switch or timer-switch capable of handling seven amps.** You may use a standard wall switch with a box and switch cover plate. Others are rocker, push button or toggle switches. I suggest using a mechanical or electronic timer-switch, although they cost about $20-50.00 more. I do not recommend a dimmer switch as they often emit strong electromagnetic fields.

- **A piece of hardware cloth or welded wire about 14-15" by 31".** This will be bent around the lamps as a guard to prevent anything from touching them.

- **Four wood screws and four 3/16" x 1" fender washers.** These are to fasten the lamp guard to the board or enclosure. You could also use a staple gun to secure the guard to the wood.

- **The board** to mount the sockets on should be about 46" high by 15" wide if you want it to sit on the floor. Alternatively, to hang the unit from the wall, the board only needs to be 12" high and 24" wide. The extra width is to mount the switch to one side of the lamps. The board can be of solid wood, masonite, veneer or plywood. For chemically sensitive people, it could be of sheet metal or hard plastic like Lucite if one is not sensitive to this material. To avoid all outgassing, use a metallic material or a poplar, oak or fir shelf board.

- **Wood screws and/or machine screws and nuts for mounting the sockets and switch to a board or enclosure.**

- **A 7-amp fuse is optional.** It is not necessary.

Tools required include a small screwdriver, wire cutters, and a drill to cut holes in the board for wires, sockets and mounting screws.

Construction

Mount the sockets to the board or enclosure in a triangle shape (see the diagram at the end of this section). If you are using a board that is 12" high by 24" wide, the top socket is placed in the center, 2" from the top of the board. The lower sockets are mounted two inches from the bottom of the board and 9.5 to 10" apart.

If you are using a board that reaches down to the floor, the top socket should be at chest height when sitting, about 36" off the floor. The two lower sockets should be mounted at abdomen height when sitting, about 28" off the floor.

Place the switch or timer-switch as far away from the lamps as possible, either to one side or above them.

Wire the sockets in *parallel* (see diagram). The lamps will not work properly if the sockets are wired in series. When wiring the sockets, one need not cut the lamp cord. It may be faster to connect two wires to one socket and then run the cord to the next socket. Separate the wires at the next socket, strip the wires just where the terminal screws are and screw down the terminals over the wires. Then continue similarly to the third socket. Run the wires to the switch. A fuse is optional.

For the protective guard in front of the lamps, bend the hardware cloth into a C shape with 1" flanges at each end. It is easiest to bend it over a sharp edge of a table or desk. Make the bends in the 31" length, so the 14-15" dimension of the hardware cloth becomes the width of the guard.

First bend the 31" piece of mesh 90° at 1". Make another 90° bend at 9", another at 22" and another at 30". Make all bends in the same direction. This should form a C shape with 1" flanges at each end for fastening to the wood with wood screws and large washers, two on the bottom and two on top. (See the diagram for details.)

To mount the board in an enclosure, you may drill holes in the corners for screws. If you will mount the electrical unit on a PVC pipe frame, you will need mounting holes for four 3/4" pipe straps.

Mounting and Ventilation. If one's unit is for a bathroom or closet, secure it to a wall so it will not fall over if accidentally bumped. In a bathroom tub area, the unit can be hung from the shower pipe. However, also tie it back so it will not move.

If you will mount it in a wooden or other enclosure, you can secure it using four wood screws, one in each corner. To mount to a PVC pipe frame, use four pipe straps.

Ventilation can be important. Most bathrooms have ventilation. In a closet, the door may not fit tightly at the top. If necessary, open the door slightly every 10 minutes or so as needed to provide ventilation. If building an enclosure, leave a 1" wide opening across the top at the front and back.

Enclosures. The electrical unit may be mounted in any suitable enclosure including a small closet, wooden box, frame enclosure or other space. If the space is larger than about 4' by 4' and 5'- 6' high, it may need an auxiliary heater or another lamp to bring the sauna to 110° F. within 20-30 minutes. For more information about enclosures, see Chapter 12.

Cautions and Disclaimer

Observe all cautions as with any electrical appliance exposed to heat and moisture. *Do not touch the lamps during use, or let water, sweat, towels or anything touch them.* Accidents can happen in saunas. Always move slowly and carefully. Never allow young children to play in or use a sauna unaccompanied. The author cannot be responsible for misuse of a sauna or poor construction.

INFRARED LIGHT SAUNA ELECTRICAL UNIT

Ceramic lamp sockets are mounted on a piece of wood 12" high by 24" wide

Be sure to wire the lamp sockets in parallel (as shown)

The hardware cloth guard over the lamps is essential

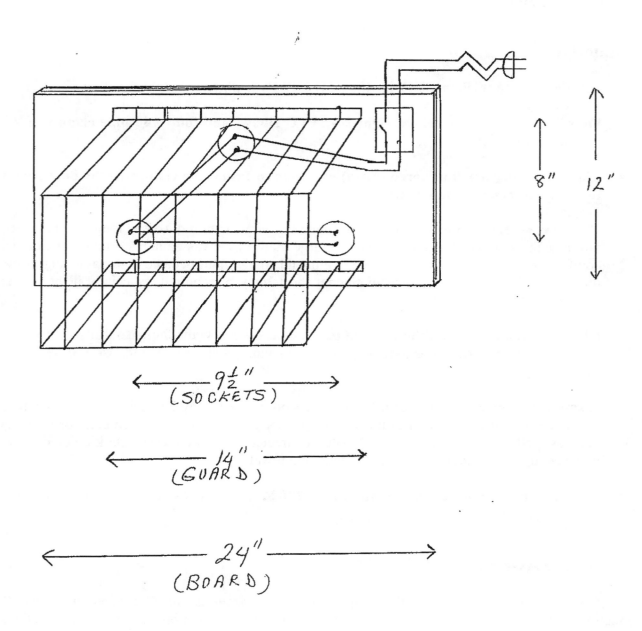

8"

12"

9½"
(SOCKETS)

14"
(GUARD)

24"
(BOARD)

Appendix E. PVC Pipe Frame Enclosure Construction Plans

An excellent inexpensive sauna enclosure consists of a frame over which one places canvas, blankets or other fabric. The frame is made of PVC pipe, although it could be made of 1"x 2" wood or other material such as steel tubing. The covering we suggest is double-layer canvas, although other fabric materials will also suffice. The total cost is usually under $100.00. Tools required are a hack saw or pipe cutter to cut PVC pipe, tape measure, screwdriver and a hammer to tap the pipe pieces together. The unit is lightweight, portable and can be easily disassembled for travel.

Materials

- **10' sticks of the thicker (SCH 40, 480 PSI) 3/4" PVC pipe.**

- **Four 3/4" PVC T-connectors, eight 3/4" PVC elbows and four 3/4" pipe clamps.** PVC cement is not needed.

- **Eight 1/2" long machine screws (#10) and nuts to fasten the clamps to the board with the lamp unit (see Appendix D).**

- **The Cover**. This can be of a variety of materials such as two queen or king-size blankets, fabric such as fleece, flannel or velour, a large cloth or canvas painter's drop cloths, quilts, comforters or flannel sheets. I do not recommend an aluminum-coated material facing inside the sauna. Two layers of canvas or flannel sheets may be required, especially if the unit is used in a cold location.

- **Clips or fasteners to hold the cover in place,** unless you sew the fabric so it fits tightly over the frame. 2" butterfly clips used as paper clasps work well. You could also use Velcro or safety pins.

- **A small stool or chair without a back.** The stool or chair may be made of wood, metal or plastic because the lower part of the sauna does not get too hot. A painted chair or bench is okay as well. Wood stools may be coated or treated with chemicals. Dark-colored metal may heat up, but could be covered with tape or a towel.

- **An outdoor thermometer that reads up to 120° F.** The best is a bimetallic type or a digital type. A fancy thermometer is not needed.

Enclosure Assembly

Pipe Assembly. Cut the PVC pipe into four 5' sections, six 4' sections and four 3" sections. Assemble as shown in the diagram that follows this section. Push the pipe sections into the connectors. Then use a hammer to gently tap the pipe firmly into the connectors. No cement should be necessary unless pipe is very loose in the connectors. The order of assembly of the sections does not matter.

Fastening the Electrical Unit. Secure the board containing the lamp sockets to the PVC frame with four 3/4" pipe clamps. Pull the two vertical frame members together where the electrical unit will attach. The frame will bend to accommodate the size of the board. In fact, this adds rigidity to the structure.

Adjust the height of the lamp unit by moving the board up or down along the vertical PVC pipe sections. Place your stool or bench inside the unit and have someone sit on it. The upper lamp should be at chest height when sitting and the lower lamps at abdomen height.

Adding the Cover. When assembly is complete, cover the frame with fabric, blankets, quilts, fleece, comforters or canvas, overlapping at the far end to create a convenient entrance. Be sure to eliminate air leaks, especially at the bottom of the enclosure. Cover the floor inside the enclosure with towels to catch any sweat that may drip during sauna use.

Screw in the three lamps and the sauna should be ready for use. Test your enclosure by mounting the thermometer at eye level and not too close to the lamps. The enclosure should heat up to 110° F. within about thirty minutes. If this does not occur, you have air leaks or more layers of insulation are needed.

Warnings and Disclaimer

Be sure to have a guard in front of the lamps and be sure fabric or blankets are 6" inches or more from the lamps to avoid a fire hazard. Pull fabric tight so it does not hang loosely near the lamps. Avoid leaving the lamps on when no one is present.

Do not allow children to play unsupervised around a sauna. If you are unsure about sauna use, always have an attendant present. Always use saunas with caution. I cannot be responsible for poor construction or misuse of your sauna enclosure.

PVC Pipe Enclosure Frame

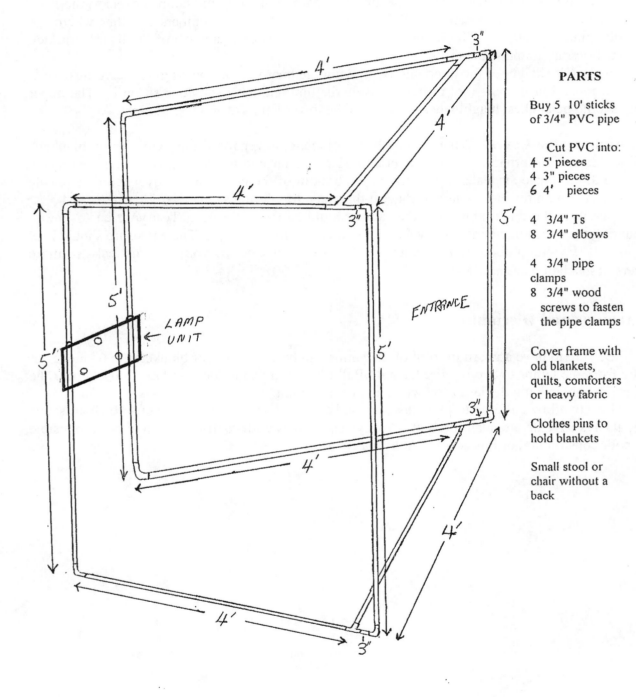

4'

4'

3"

4'

4'

5'

5'

5'

3"

LAMP UNIT

ENTRANCE

5'

4'

3"

4'

4'

3"

PARTS

Buy 5 10' sticks of 3/4" PVC pipe

Cut PVC into:
4 5' pieces
4 3" pieces
6 4' pieces

4 3/4" Ts
8 3/4" elbows

4 3/4" pipe clamps
8 3/4" wood screws to fasten the pipe clamps

Cover frame with old blankets, quilts, comforters or heavy fabric

Clothes pins to hold blankets

Small stool or chair without a back

148

Appendix F.   Benefits of An Single Reddish Heat Lamp

A single reddish heat lamp directed at an area of the body provides excellent and often surprising benefits. Infrared energy heats several inches deep, improving the circulation and disabling microorganisms. Single lamp therapy, in our experience, is simple, inexpensive and very safe when properly handled.

Conditions that may benefit, often after just a few treatments, include *joint pain, muscle strains, skin rashes, acne, boils* and some conditions of the *eyes, nose, ears* and *sinuses. Neck, shoulder, elbow, knee* and *back pain* may also respond.

One patient had a sinus infection that did not respond to antibiotics or to natural healing methods. She was weak and feverish every evening and had constant headaches. By shining an infrared lamp on the sinuses for 10 minutes at a time, six times a day, relief occurred in two days with complete elimination of all symptoms in five days. The patient continued to use the lamp for another two weeks because she said the red light felt wonderful.

Relief in one or two days has also occurred in cases of low back pain, knee pain, nerve root irritation and other local conditions. One can safely shine the lamp on any area of the body in need of healing.

Those who may not use a sauna such as pregnant and lactating women, and young children can safely benefit from a single lamp. It can also be used on pets and large animals such as horses. Do not place a pet in a sauna, as animals can easily overheat.

Single Lamp Protocol

Purchase a 250-watt, **reddish,** incandescent "heat lamp". Do not use a clear bulb, but the bulb need not be pure red. Also purchase a clamp-on lamp socket rated for at least a 250-watt light bulb. Both of these are inexpensive and sold in many hardware stores. One could also use an adjustable lamp in the home for the bulb. It, too, should be rated for a 250-watt bulb.

For the head area, such as sinuses, ears or teeth: Use the lamp for five to ten minutes per session, up to six or seven times per day. *Do not use it longer than 10 minutes at a time.*

For the rest of the body: Use the lamp for ten to sixty minutes per session, and you may do two or three sessions each day.

One sits about 12" to 24" from the lamp and moves the lamp around the area during the treatment. Allow the area to become as hot as one can comfortably tolerate.   If the lamp is fixed, move the body slightly. Remaining in one spot for a few moments causes a slight reddening of the skin that will go away quickly and is not harmful. Remaining in one spot too long, however, could cause a serious burn.

A simple way to do therapy is to clamp the lamp socket to a shelf and sit comfortably near the lamp so that it shines on the desired part of the body without causing strain.

Cautions With A Single Infrared Lamp

Move the lamp back and forth slightly or move the body part it is directed toward. Close the eyes when directing the lamp at the eyes, nose or sinuses. *Avoid* using the lamp on an injury for the first 24 hours following the injury.

Avoid shining the lamp at the head for more than 10 minutes at a time.
Avoid touching a heat lamp when it is hot.
Avoid placing the bulb on any surface when hot to avoid igniting or burning the surface.
Avoid banging the lamp or splashing water on it, as these could cause it to break.

Other Infrared Therapy Systems

Battery-operated LED Lamps. Many companies sell infrared therapy devices using light-emitting diodes (LEDs). These vary in their penetrating power and offer some of the same benefits as the 250-watt infrared lamp. However, they are usually much less powerful.

Infrared Clothing. Thermoflow Company, and perhaps several others, offer underclothing that contains special material that, when heated by body heat, emits infrared frequencies. Silk clothing also does this, to some extent. However, this is not nearly the same as near infrared sauna therapy.

Sunbathing As Infrared Therapy. Many people ask if they can just sunbathe to obtain the same benefits as sauna therapy. I wish this were true, but it is not. The sun contains many frequencies of light and radiation, some of which are harmful. Also, sweating does not occur as well during sunbathing as with a near infrared lamp sauna. Overall, the effect is not the same.

GLOSSARY

Aldosterone	Hormone which acts on the kidneys to regulate the level of salt and water in the blood
Angiogenesis	The formation of blood vessels
Apoptosis	Programmed cell death
Ascites	The abnormal accumulation of serous fluid in the abdominal cavity
Bile	A bitter greenish-yellow liquid secreted by the liver and stored in the gall bladder - it aids digestion in the small intestine by neutralizing acids and emulsifying fats
Borrelia burgdorferi	Bacteria which causes Lyme disease (see below)
Bovine	To do with cattle
Bradykinin	A powerful vasodilator found in blood plasma
Catalase	An enzyme present in most human cells
Chakras	The seven body centers or sites viewed in certain forms of yoga as sources of psychic or spiritual energy
Chi	Chinese word for energy or vital force; vital energy that is held to animate the body internally and is of central importance in some Eastern systems of medical treatment (as acupuncture) and of exercise or self-defense (as tai chi)
Cholecystitis	Inflammation of the gall bladder
Choline	Constituent of vitamin B complex - prevents accumulation of fat in the liver
Cholinesterase	An enzyme found in blood plasma and in the liver
Conduction (sauna)	Heats the body by direct contact with steam or hot sand; in physics conduction is the transmission of electricity, heat, etc. through a material
Congestive heart failure	Chronic inability of the heart to maintain an adequate output of blood resulting in congestion and over-distension of certain veins and organs with blood and correspondingly an inadequate blood supply to other body tissues

Conjugates	In biochemistry to say something is conjugating is to say it's undergoing chemical change
Convection (sauna)	Moves hot air around the body; in physics convection is the transfer of heat from one place to another by the circulation of currents of heated particles of a gas or liquid
Dehydrocholic acid	Cholagogue: a drug which causes an increased flow of bile into the intestine
Denaturation	A usually irreversible alteration of the native structure of a protein, for example, the beating and scrambling of eggs
Divertculosis	An intestinal disorder characterized by the presence of numerous diverticula (abnormal pouches or sac openings in the intestine or bladder)
Diverticulitis	Inflammation of a diverticulum (pouch or sac in the intestine)
DMPS	Chelator of heavy metals used as a provoking agent in testing for the presence of heavy metals and as a treating agent for heavy metal toxicity
DMSA	Dimercaptosuccinic Acid (DMSA), a non-toxic, water-soluble treatment for heavy metal toxicity
Dysbiosis	*Dysbiosis* means there is too much yeast, harmful bacteria, viruses or parasites in the intestines
EDTA	A white crystalline acid used especially as a chelating agent, a preservative, and in medicine as an anticoagulant and in the treatment of lead poisoning
Electrolytes	Minerals dissolved or suspended in solution which create an electrical charge that is needed energy for the body to function. They help maintain stable blood pressure and circulation, regulate body temperature, transport nutrients, detoxify metabolic waste (heavy metals, toxic chemicals, etc.) and lubricate musculoskeletal joints; including such minerals as sodium, potassium, and magnesium
Electron transport system	A key part of the energy production system occurring in metabolism
Endotoxins	A toxic product of bacteria which is associated with the structure of the cell and can only be obtained by destruction of the cell (see exotoxin)
Eosinophils	A white blood cell that is present at sites of allergic reactions and parasitic infections
Epinephrine	A hormone secreted by the adrenal gland; also known as adrenaline, part of the fight or flight sympathetic nervous system, vasoconstrictor and heart stimulant
Epitopes	Surface characteristics of cancer cells that allow the immune system to identify it as dangerous

Erysipelas	Bacterial infection of the skin and tissues beneath the skin giving a characteristic reddened sharply outlined appearance, accompanied by high fever and marked toxic reaction
Etheric	Ethereal
Exotoxin	A toxic product of bacterial which is passed into the environment of the cell during growth - opposite of endotoxin (see endotoxin)
Ferric	Of, relating to, or containing iron (see ferrous)
Ferrous	Of, relating to, or containing iron (as distinguished from ferric). "Ferric" and "ferrous" describe two different forms of iron
GABA	gamma-aminobutyric acid; a powerful amino acid that is classified as a neurotransmitter, which means it helps nerve impulses bridge the gaps between synapses and communicate better
Glucuronides	A product of glucose metabolism which is excreted in urine
Glutathione	An amino acid that plays a role in basic biochemical reactions
Glycolysis	The process by which a carbohydrate such as glucose is broken down into an acid as part of the sequence of producing cellular energy
Heat shock proteins	Heating the body can temporarily suspend synthesis of normal body proteins and instead induce production of special proteins that preserve and restore normal cell activity. These heat shock proteins enhance the immune system and improve cellular energy production, respiration, elimination and other cell functions
HSPs	See heat shock proteins
Hydrochloric acid	An aqueous solution of hydrogen chloride (HCl), a strong corrosive irritating acid normally present in dilute form in gastric juice, and widely used in industry and in the laboratory
Hypothalamus	A region of the pain that sits under the thalamus controlling temperature, hunger, thirst, the pituitary gland, etc.
Inositol	A part of Vitamin B complex
ischemia	Deficient supply of blood to a body part (as the heart or brain) due to an obstruction in blood flow
Kelp	Any of various large brown seaweed
Liver	The large, reddish-brown organ in vertebrate animals that secretes bile and is active in the absorption and storage of vitamins, minerals, and sugar (which it changes into glycogen). The liver frees the blood of its waste matter and manufactures blood proteins; principal

	detoxification organ of the body.
Kreb's cycle	Cycle of intracellular chemical reactions by means of which organisms convert food chemicals into physical energy (named after Sir Hans A. Krebs, 1900 - 1981, an English biochemist who discovered it)
Lyme disease	A condition thought to be transmitted through the bite of a tick, characterized by a ring-shaped rash surrounding the bite area and attacks of recurring arthritis
Lymphocytes	Any of several white blood cells found in the lymph nodes, in the spleen, and in the blood, which are agents of the immune system and constitute 20 to 30 percent of the white blood cells of normal human blood
Micron	Micrometer: a unit of length equal to one millionth of a meter also called a micron
Mitochochondria	See mitochondria
Mitochondria	Any of various round or long structures that are found outside the nucleus of the cell, and produce energy for the cell through cellular respiration, and are rich in fats, proteins, and enzymes
Nanometer	One billionth of a meter
Nettles	Any of a group of herbs having sharp hairs on the leaves and stems that sting the skin when touched and possessing medicinal properties
Niacin	A part of vitamin B complex
Norepinephrine	A crystalline compound that occurs as a hormone with epinephrine and that has a strong vasoconstrictor action and mediates transmission of sympathetic nerve impulses but lacks or exhibits weakly most other epinephrine effects; also known as noradrenalin
Pancreatin	A mixture of enzymes from pancreatic juice; also a preparation extracted from the pancreas of animals, used to aid digestion
Parasympathetic nervous system	Opposite of the sympathetic nervous system; that part of the autonomic (involuntary) nervous system that produces such involuntary responses as dilating blood vessels, increasing the activity of digestion and reproductive organs and glands and slowing down heartbeat
Preoptic	Situated in front of an optic part or region such as preoptic tracts in the brain
Prion	A protein particle lacking a nucleic acid and implicated in various neuro-generative diseases
Radiant (sauna)	Uses heat rays generated by ceramic far infrared elements, electric light bulbs or by the sun; energy traveling as electromagnetic waves
Renaturation	Reconstitution of damaged proteins

Scrapie	Virus disease of sheep and goats
Seratia marcescens	Type of bacteria
Serous fluid	A discharge of material resembling the serum of blood
Silymarin	Silymarin refers to the extract from the seeds of the plant *Silybum marianum*, also called "milk thistle". It has been used for over 2,000 years as a liver tonic. The active ingredients of milk thistle are silybin, silydianin, and silychristin, collectively known as *silymarin*
Spirochetes	A kind of bacteria, one type of which causes syphilis
Spongiform	Sponge-like
Streptococcus pyogenes	Type of bacteria
Sympathetic nervous system	That part of the autonomic nervous system that involves the fight or flight mechanism, increasing heartbeat, vaso-constriction and blood pressure, etc. Opposite to the parasympathetic system.
T-cell	Any of several lymphocytes (a type of white blood cells) matured in the thymus (hence T cell) which destroy foreign proteins and stimulate antibody production.
Telomeres	Protein fragments that, according to recent research attach themselves to DNA and are a factor in aging
Thalamus	A part of the brain involved with perception
Theophylline	A bitter crystalline compound extracted from tea leaves but usually made synthetically, and closely related to caffeine, that is used in medicine often in the form of derivatives or combinations with other drugs chiefly as a muscle relaxant in asthma, as a vasodilator, and as a diuretic
Thymus	A small ductless glandlike organ found in young vertebrates near the base of the neck and disappearing or becoming rudimentary in the adult, which functions as an organ of the immune system involved in the maturation of T cells.
Totipotent	Capable of development along any of the lines inherently possible to its kind
Transcription	A step in the process whereby DNA is transcribed or copied so its information can be relayed on a cellular level
Ureter	A duct that conveys urine from a kidney to the bladder
Zirconium	A white metallic element used in alloys for wires and filaments, etc.; a form of zirconium is used for making artificial gems

RESOURCES

NEAR INFRARED LAMP SAUNAS

Parts And Complete Near Infrared Sauna Units. Please visit **www.drlwilson.com.** Click on the link near the top of the home page that reads "Find Someone To build You A Near Infrared Sauna".

OTHER PRODUCTS AND SERVICES

Hair Tissue Mineral Analysis. For a current list of practitioners who offer this service in the specific way that Dr. Paul Eck used the test, with the latest research, please visit **www.drlwilson.com.** Click on the link on the home page that reads something like "How To Find A Nutritional Balancing Practitioner. *These are the only practitioners I can recommend.*

Color Therapy. An excellent organization is the Dinshaw Health Society, PO Box 707, Malaga, NJ USA 08328, (856)-692-4686. They offer books and color therapy products based on the work of Dinshaw Ghadiali, a pioneer of color therapy.

Realmilk.com - This website may help you find local sources of raw dairy products.

Corrections And Updates For This Book. Please check the website, **www.drlwilson.com,** for corrections and updates for this book (the 2014 edition).

References

Books

Aaland, M., *Sweat*, Capra Press, 1978.

Beard, J. *The Enzyme Treatment of Cancer*, London, Chatto and Windus, 1911.

Cowen, T. and McGuire, J., *Spas & Hot Tubs, Saunas and Home Gyms*, Creative Homeowner Press, Upper Saddle River, NJ, 1988.

Casdorph, H.R. and Walker, M., *Toxic Metal Syndrome*, Avery Publishing Group, NY, 1995.

Dennis, C., *Colorology*, Rainbows Unlimited, Clearwater, FL, 1994.

Dinshaw, D., *Let There Be Light*, Dinshaw Health Society, Malaga, NJ, 2005.
Douglas, W.C., *Into the Light*, Second Opinion Publishing, Dunwoody, GA, 1993.

Dreosti, I.E. and Smith, R.M., ed., *Neurobiology of the Trace Elements, Vol. 1 & 2,* The Humana Press, NJ, 1983.

Flickstein, A., *Infrared Thermal System for Whole-body Regenerative Radiant Therapy*, Dascom Graphics, Santa Fe Springs, 1997.

Finnish Medical Society, *Sauna and Your Health: Annals of Clinical Research*, 16 technical articles distributed by the Sauna Society of America, 1988.

Finnish Sauna Society, *Sauna Studies*, professional papers from the 6th International Sauna Congress of 1974, distributed by the Sauna Society of America.
Gerson, M., *A Cancer Therapy - Results of 50 Cases*, Totality Books, CA, 1958,1977.

Ghadiali, D., *Spectro-Chome Metry Encyclopedia*, Dinshaw Health Society, Malaga, NJ, 1933.

Ghadiali, D., *History of Spectro-Chrome*, Dinshaw Health Society, Malaga, NJ, 1957.

Guyton, A., *Textbook of Medical Physiology*, 6th edition, W. B. Saunders Company, 1981.

Hollander, C., *How to Build a Sauna*, Drake, New York, 1978.

Hubbard, L.R., *Clear Body, Clear Mind*, Bridge Publications, Los Angeles, Ca., 2002.

Jensen, B., *Doctor-Patient Handbook*, BiWorld Publishers, Inc., UT, 1976.

Johnson, T. and Miller, T., *The Sauna Book*, Harper and Row, New York, 1977.

Kaufmann, S.H.F., ed, *Heat Shock Proteins and the Immune Response*, Springer Publishing, 1991.

Kervan, L.C., *Biological Transmutations*, adapted by Michel Abehsera, Swan House Publishing, Binghampton, NY, 1972. (Now published by Beekman Publishers, Inc, Woodstock, NY)

Koch, W.F., *The Survival Factor in Neoplastic and Viral Diseases*, William F. Koch, 1961.

Kukreja, R.C., ed., *Heat Shock Proteins in Myocardial Protection*, Landes Bioscience, 2000.

Kutsky, R., *Handbook of Vitamins, Minerals and Hormones*, 2nd edition, Van Nostrand Reinhold, 1981.

Lehmann, J.F., *Therapeutic Heat and Cold*, 4th ed., Lippincott, Williams and Wilkins, 1990.

McVicker, M., *Sauna Detoxification Therapy*, McFarland & Co., Jefferson, NC, 1997.

Nover, L., ed, *The Heat Shock Response*, CRC Press, 1991.

Pfeiffer, C., *Mental and Elemental Nutrients*, Keats Publishing, New Canaan CT, 1975.

Rogers, S.A., *Tired or Toxic*, Prestige Publishers, 1990. (Also *Detoxify or Die*, 2002)

Roy, R., *The Sauna*, Chelsea Green Publishing Company, White River Junction, VT, 1996.

Sylver, N., *Holistic Handbook of Sauna Therapy*, The Center For Frequency, Stone Ridge, NY 2004.

Takada, K., Egawa, Y., Sasaki, H., *Far Infrared Rays,* Japan, 1999.

Verlag, S., *Heat Shock*, 1991.

Viherjuuri, H.J., *Sauna: The Finnish Bath*, The Stephen Green Press, Brattleboro, VT, 1965.

Wilson, L., *Nutritional Balancing and Hair Mineral Analysis*, L.D. Wilson Consultants, Inc., 2005.

Yamazaki, T., *Science of Far Infrared Wave Therapies*, Man and History Co., Tokyo, Japan, 1987.

Articles

Ahonen, E., et al, 1988, Fluid balance and the sauna, *Duodecin.*, 104(8):609-14.

Antonachi, F., et al.,1998, Sweating patterns in humans: II. Heat-induced forehand sweating and cutaneous temperature in healthy individuals, *Funct Neurol.*, 3(2)(Apr-Jun):2217-24.

Badermann, E., 1976, Aesthetic and physiological sensory perceptions in the original Finnish sauna, *Sauna Studies,* Papers read at the VI International Sauna Congress in Helsinki, August 15-17, 1974. The Finnish Sauna Society, Helsinki.

Baibekov, I.M., et al., 1994, The effects of low intensity infrared laser radiation on healing of dermatological wounds, *Bull Eksp Biol Med.,* 119(2)(Feb):218-24.

Beard, J., 1902, Embriological aspects and the etiology of carcinoma, *The Lancet,* 1:1758.

Cherniaev, I.S., 1965, Investigation of the permeability of human skin to infrared radiation, *Gig Sanit.,* 30(12)(Dec):20-24.

Chlamydial Heat Shock Proteins in Severe Disease, Dec. 2002, MEW, www.chalmydiae.com/chlamydiae/docs/biology/hsp

Cohn, J.R. and E.A. Emmett, 1978, The excretion of trace metals in human sweat, *Ann Clin and Lab Sci.,* 8(4):270-274.

Coley, W.B., A Preliminary Note on the Treatment of Inoperable Sarcoma by the Toxic Product of Erysipelas, *Post-Graduate Med.,* 8:278-86, 1893.

Czarnowski, D.J., J. Gorski et al., 1991, Excretion of nitrogen compounds in sweat during sauna, *Pol Tyg Lek.,* 46(8-10)(Feb. 18-Mar 4):186-187.

Danno, K. and N. Sugie, 1996, Effects of near-infrared radiation on the epidermal proliferation and cutaneous immune function in mice, *Photodermal Photoimmuniol Photomed,* 12(6)(Dec):233-6.

Didierjean, L., D. Gruaz, Y. Frober, J.Grassi, J.M. Dayer, J.H. Saurat, 1990, Biologically active interleukin in human eccrine sweat: site dependent variations in alpha/beta ratios and stress-induced increased excretion, *Cytokine.,*2(6)(Nov):438-46.

Dritschilo, A., et al., 1981, Therapeutic implication of heat as related to radiation therapy, *Semin Oncol.,* 8(1)(March):83-91.

Eck, P., 1981, A beginning course on energy and minerals, *Healthview Newsletter,* (27-29):1-44. Eck Institute of Applied Nutrition and Bioenergetics, Ltd.

Eells, J.T.et al, 2003, Therapeutic photobiomodulation for methanol-induced retinal toxicity, *Proc Natl Acad of Sci.,* doi:10.1073/pnas.05347461000, March 7.

Enwemeka, C.S., Therapeutic Light, *Interdiscipl. J. of Rehab.,* Jan/Feb 2004.

Ernst, E., P. Wirz, T. Saradeth, 1990, Regular sauna bathing and the incidence of common colds, *Ann Med.,* 22(4):225-7.

Flickstein, A., 2000, Healthmate infrared saunas, *Townsend Letter for Doctors*, 202(May):66-70.

Gard, Z.R. and E.J. Brown, 1992-1999, History of sauna/hyperthermia; Past and present efficacy in detoxification, *Townsend Letter for Doctors*, June 1992:470-478, July 1992:650-660, Oct. 1992:846-854, Aug-Sept 1999:76-86.

Goncalves, E., 2001, The secret nuclear war, *The Ecologist*, 31(3)April:28-33.

Graeffe, G., et al., 1996, The ions in sauna air, *Sauna Studies*, Papers read at the VI International Sauna Congress in Helsinki, August 15-17, 1974. The Finnish Sauna Society, Helsinki.

Gumener, P.I., O.V. Kaisina, L.G. Nadezhina, T.V. Shumkova, 1994,The individual measuring of the health-promoting impact of the sauna on preschoolers, *Vopr Kurortol Fizioter Lech Fix Kult*, (5)(Sept-Oct):32-5.

"Heat Shock Proteins: New Avenue to Cancer Vaccines", *Cancer Research Institute*, New York, 2002.

Helamaa, E. and E. Aikas, 1988, The secret of good 'loyly', *Ann Clin Res.*, 20(4):224-9.

Honda, K. and S. Inoue, 1988, Sleep-enhancing effects of far infrared radiation in rats, *Int J Biometeorol.*, 32(2)(June):92-4.

Hrnjak, M., 1985, The effect of infrared irradiation on the human body, *Arh Hig Rada Toksikol.*, 36(2)(June):201-18.

Ikeda, Y. and C. Tei, 2002, Effect of repeated sauna therapy on survival of TO-2 cardiomyopathic hampsters with heart failure, *Am J Cardiology*, 90(Aug 1):343-345.

Inoue, S. and M. Kabaya, 1989, Biological activities caused by far infrared radiation, *Int J Biometeorol*, 33(3)(Oct):145-50.

Ise, N., T. Katsuura, Y. Kikuchi and E. Miwa, 1987, Effect of far-infrared radiation on forearm skin blood flow, *Ann Physiol Anthropol.*, 6(1)(Jan):31-32.

Jenssen, T.G., H.H. Haukland, P.G. Burhol, 1988, Brain-gut peptides in sauna-induced hyperthermia, *Acta Physiol Scand.*, 132(4)(April):519-523.

Jezova, D., R. Kvetnansky, M. Vigas, 1994, Sex differences in endocrine response to hyperthermia in sauna, *Acta Physiol Scand.*, 150(3)(March):293-298.

Jiang, P. and L. Luo, 1997, The effect of far infrared rays on the survival of randomized skin flap in the rat: an experimental study, *Chung Kuo Hsiu Fu Chung Chien Wai Ko Tsa Chih.*, 11(2)(March):69-71.

Jokinen, E., I. Valimaki, J. Marniemi, A. Seppanen, K. Irjala, O. Simell, 1991, Children in sauna: hormonal adjustments to intensive short thermal stress, *Acta Physiol Scand.*, 142(3)(July):437-442.

Junaid, A.J., 1986, Treatment of cutaneous leishmaniasis with infrared heat, *Int J Dermatol.*, 25(7)(Sept):470-2.

Jurasunas, S., 2000, A far-infrared ray emitting stone (SGES) to treat cancer and degenerative diseases, *Townsend Letter for Doctors*, 203(June):123-134.

Kaderavek, R., 1965, Thermoregulatory changes during application of infrared radiation, *Fysiatr Revmatol Vestn.*, 43(5)(Sept):301-9.

Kaderavek, R., 1971, Absorption and heat transport during application of infrared radiation, *Fysiatr Revmatol Vestn.*, 51(1)(Feb):14-20.

Kaidbey, K.H., et al., 1982, The influence of infrared radiation on short-term ultraviolet-radiation-induced injuries, *Arch Dermatol.*, 118(5)(May):315-18.

Kauppinen, K., et al., 1986, Man in the sauna, *Ann Clin Res.*, 18(4):173-185.

Khish, I.P., 1973, Effect of low doses of infrared radiation on the sympathetic-adrenal system of children, *Pediatr Akush Ginekol.*, 6:23-24.

Kihara, T., et al., 2002, Repeated sauna treatment improves vascular endothelial and cardiac function in patients with chronic heart failure, *J Am Coll of Cardiology*, 39(March 6):754-759.

Kihara, T. et al, 2002, Sauna therapy decreases cardiac arrhymias in patients with chronic heart failure, *Am Heart Assn Scientific Sessions*, Nov. 17-20, Chicago.

Kilburn, K.H., R. H. Warsaw, M.G. Shields, 1989, Neurobehavioral dysfunction in firemen exposed to polychlorinated biphenyls (PCBs):possible improvement after detoxification, *Arch Environ Health*, 44(6)(Nov-Dec):345-50.

Krop, J. and J. Swierczek, 1987/1988, Patient with severe intractable asthma, urticaria and irritable bowel syndrome: Response to sauna therapy, *Clin Ecology*, 5:136-139.

Krop, J., 1998, Chemical sensitivity after intoxication at work with solvents: response to sauna therapy, *J Altern Complementary Med.*, 4(1)(Spring):77-86.

Kukkonen-Jarjula, K., and K. Jkauppinen, 1998, How the sauna affects the endocrine system, *Ann Clin Res.*, 20(4):262-6.

Libert, J.P., et al., 1983, Modifications of sweating responses to thermal transients following heat acclimation, *Eur J Appl Physiol.*, 50(2):235-46.

Linetskii, M.L., 1965, Thermoregulation under the effect of infrared radiation, *Gig Sanit.*,30(7)(July):115-17.

Lovejoy, H.B., Z.G. Bell, T.R. Vizena, 1973, Mercury exposure evaluations and their correlation with urine mercury excretion: 4. Elimination of mercury by sweating, *J Occup Med.,*15:590-591.

Marler, M.S., et al., Overexpression of the rat inducible 70-KD heat stress protein in a transgenic mouse increases the resistance of the heart to ischemic injury, 1995, *J Clin Investigation*, 95:1446-56.
Marmor, J.B.,et al., 1980, Combined radiation and hyperthermia in superficial human tumors, *Cancer*, 46(9)(Nov 1):1986-91.

Martin, W., 2003, Coley's toxins for sarcoma and intractable cancer, *Townsend Letter for Doctors*, #235-236, (Feb/March):140-144.

McCluggage, D., 1971, The sauna experience, *American Home*, February.

Molchanov, I.S., 1968, The effects of low intensity infrared radiation on the organism, *Gig Tr Prof Zabol.*, 12(11)(Nov):46-48.

Molchanov, I.S., et al., 1976, Use of low-intensity infrared radiation for the prevention of catarrhal diseases, *Gig Tr Prof Zabol.*, 9(Sept):42-43.

Moss, R., The War on Cancer, *The Townsend Letter*, #240, July 2003, pp.34-35.

Musin, R.F., et al., 1986, Sensitivity of human skin to infrared heat fluxes, *Doki Akad Nauk SSSR.*, 289(3):718-20.

Cadmium Mimics Estrogen, Nature, August 2003.

National Aeronautics And Space Administration, Light Emitting Diodes Bring Relief to Young Cancer Patients, 11/26/03. from www.nasa.gov/vision/earth/technologies/led_treatment.

Niwa, Y., O. Lizawa, K. Ishimoto, X. Jiang, T, Kanoh, 1993, Electromagnetic wave emitting products and 'Kikoh' potentiate human leukocyte functions, *Int J Biometeorol.*, 37(5)(Sept):133-8.

Niwa, Y., *1996, Jap J of Inflamm.*, 16(6)(Nov):4-9. (mechanisms of infrared-emitting stones)

Null, G. and M. Feldman, 2002, The fluoride controversy continues, parts 1,2 & 3, *Townsend Letter for Doctors*, #233, 234, 235(Dec., Jan., Feb.).
Ogita, S., et. al., 1990, Effects of far infrared radiation on lactation, *Ann Physiol Anthropol.*, 9(2)(April):83-91.

Oosterveld, F.G.J., J.J. Rasker, M.A.F. Van de Laar, and G.J. Koel, Clinical effects of infrared whole-body hyperthermia in patients with rheumatic diseases, Departments of Rheumatology and Physiotherapy, Metisch Spectrum Twente and Univeristy Twente Enschede, PO Box 50000, 7500 KA Eschede, The Netherlands.

Parpalei, I.A., L.G. Prokofeva and V.G. Obertas, 1991, The use of the sauna for disease prevention in the workers of enterprises with chemical and physical occupational hazards, *Vrach Delo.*, 5(May):93-5.

Rea, W.J., 1997, Thermal chamber depuration and physical therapy, *Chemical Sensitivity,* CRC Presss, Boca Raton, Fl, Vol. 4, Chap. 35, pp. 2433-2479.

Rea, W.J., Y. Pan, A.R. Johnson, 1991, Clearing of toxic volatile hydrocarbons from humans, *Bol Asoc Med P R*, 83(7)(July):321-4.

Rea, W.J., G.H. Ross, A.R. Johnson, R.E. Amiley, E.J. Fenyes, 1991, Chemical sensitivity in physicians, *Bol Asoc Med P R*, 83(9)(Sept):383-8.

Roehm, D.C., 1983, Effects of a program of sauna baths and metavitamins on adipose DDE and PCBs and on clearing of symptoms of agent orange (Dioxin) toxicity, *Clin Research*, 31(2):243.

Root, D.E. and G.T. Lionelli, 1987, Excretion of a lipophilic toxicant through the sebaceous glands: A case report, *J Toxicol.*, 6(1):13-17.

Schnare, D.W., M. Ben and M.G. Shields, 1984, Body burden reductions of PCBs, PBBs and chlorinated pesticides in human subjects, *Ambio* 13(5-6):378-380.

Schnare, D.W., G. Genk, M.G. Shields and S. Brunton, 1982, Evaluation of a detoxification regimen for fat stored xenobiotics, *Med Hypoth.*, 9:265-82.

Schnare, D.W. and P.C. Robinson, 1985, Reduction of hexachlorobenzene and ployclorinated biphenyl human body burdens, *Int. Agency for Research on Cancer*, WHO, Scientific Publication Series, Vol. 77, Oxford University Press.

Sealre, A.J., 1982, Effects of the sauna, *JAMA*, 247(1)(Jan 1):28.

Sherson, D.L. and W. Stopford, 1986, Mercury levels in sweat. Its use in the diagnosis and treatment of poisoning, *Ugeskr Laeger.,* 148(27)(June 30):1682-4.

Siewert, C., H. Siewert, H.J. Winterfield and D. Strangefield, 1994, The behavior of central and peripheral hemodynamics in isometric and dynamic stress in hypertensive patients: treatment with regular sauna therapy, *Z Kardiol.,* 83(9)(Sept):652-7.

Sorri, P., 1988, The sauna and sauna bathing habits: A psychoanalytic point of view, *Ann Clin Res.*, 20(4).

Strbak, V., P. Tatr, R. Angyal, V. Strec, K. Aksamitova, M. Vigas, H. Janosova, 1987, Effects of sauna and glucose intake on TSH and thyroid hormone levels in plasma of euthyroid subjects, *Metabolism*, 36(5)(May):426-31.

Tamura, Y., et al., 1997, Immunotherapy of tumors with autologous tumor-derived heat shock protein preparations, *Science*, 278:117-120.

Tei, C., Y, Horikiri, J.C. Park, J.W. Jeong, R.S. Chang, Y. Toyama, N. Tanaka, 1994, Effects of hot water bath or sauna on patients with congestive heart failure: acute hemodynamic improvement by thermal vasodilation, *J Cardiol.*, 24(3)(May-June):175-83.

Vaha-Eskeli, K. and R. Ekkola, 1988, The sauna and pregnancy, *Ann Clin Res.*, 20(4).

Vanakoski, J. and T. Seppala, 1997, Renal excretion of tetracycline is transiently decreased during short-term heat exposure, *Int J Clin Parmacol Therapy*, 35(5)(May):204-7.

Varanovski, I.M., 1967, On the use of infrared techniques in medicine, *Voen Med Zh.*, 12:36-9.

Vescovi, P.P., and V.Coiro, 1993, Hyperthermia and endorphins, *Biomed Pharmacother*, 47(8):301-4.

Vuori, I., 1988, Healthy and unhealthy sauna bathing, *Ann Clin Res.*, 20(4).

Wiedemann, E., 1965, Heat as a remedy, *Landarzt*, 44(32)(Nov 20):1586-90.

Winterfield, H.G, H. Siewert, D. Strangefield, H. Warnke, J. Kruse, U. Engelmann, 1992, Potential use of the sauna in the long-term treatment of hypertensive cardiovascular circulation disorders - a comparison with kinesiotherapy, *Schweiz Rundsch Med Prax.*, 81(35)(Aug 25):1016-20.

Wyss, V., 1966, On the effects of radiant heat on different regions of the human body. Behavior of cardiocirculatory and respiratory activity, oxygen consumption, oral and skin temperature during infrared radiation of different areas in acclimatized and non-acclimatized subjects, *Med Lav.*, 57(4)(April):262-85.

Ylikahri, R., E. Heikkonen and A. Suokas, 1988, The sauna and alcohol, *Ann Clin Res.*, (20)4.

Zelentsova, S.P., 1968, Immunobiological reactivity of the organism under the effect of the interrupted infrared irradiation, *Varach Delo.*, 12(Dec):88-91.

Zelentsova, S.P., 1970, The effects of intermittent infrared radiation on the status of natural immunological reactivity of workers *Gig Tr Prof Zabol.* 14(1)(Jan):22-6.

INDEX

acclimatization to sweating, 11
aches and pains, 118
acne, 19, 72, 149
acupuncture meridians, heating, 20
acute infections, 36, 78
addiction, 70
adhesions, 73
AIDS, 69
alcohol, 39
alkalinity, 45
aluminum, 4
antagonists, 47
anti-aging therapy, 7
anxiety, 95
aromatherapy, 54
arsenic, 5, 121
arteriosclerosis, 70
arthritis, 27
ascites, 87
atherosclerosis, 70
attitudes
    healing, 66
bacteria, 13
Beard, J., MD, 81
bed rest, 78
biological toxins, 5
biological transmutation, 33
body position, 105
body temperature
    increased, 13
    low, 14
breakfast suggestions, 64
breathing, conscious, 54
burns, 72
bursitis, 72
cabinets, 99
cadmium, 4
calcium, 5, 121
calories, burning, 20

cancer, 13, 23, 81
    definition, 81
    intestinal, 73
    protocol, 87
    sauna benefits, 81
    sauna mechanisms, 85
candida albicans, 41, 73
cardiovascular benefits, 69
cardiovascular effects, 18
cardiovascular rehabilitation, 70
catalase, 25
cautions with saunas, 36
charcoal tablets, 59
chelation, 47
chemical exposure, 71
chemicals, toxic, 3, 13
children, 38
chlorine, 4
cholecystitis, 73
chromium, 5, 121
chronic fatigue, 73
chronic fatigue syndrome, 41
chronic infections, 79
circulation, enhanced, 14, 17, 44, 76
claims, untrue, 15
claustrophobia, 29, 40
cluster chains, shortening, 16
cold plunges, 58
Coley, W., MD, 26, 85
Coley's toxins, 26
colitis, 19, 73
color therapy, 17, 56, 77, 87
computer sensitivity, 119
condiments and snacks, 63
conduction, 97
congestive heart failure, 70
connective tissue disorders, 72

constipation, 73, 118
convection, 97
converting saunas, 109
cooking, 64
cool bathing, 58
copper, 5
cortisol, 77
cows milk, 62
damaged DNA, 13
dandruff, 72
danger signals, 40
deep tissue heating, 15
deep tissue penetration, 45
defective cells, 13
density concept, 50
dental abscess, 89
dental amalgams, 88
dermatitis, 19
detoxification, 41
detoxification ability, 134
detoxification difficulties, 51
detoxification mechanisms, 42
detoxification programs, 126
diabetes, 37
diarrhea, 73, 95, 119
diet, 61
digestive disorders, 73
digestive system effects, 19
disclaimer statement, 141
diverticulitis, 73
diverticulosis, 73
DNA, 14
drug detoxification, 70
dysbiosis, 73
ear infections, 72
eating habits, 64
eating out, 63
Eck, Dr. P.C., vi

eczema, 19, 72
edema, 14, 72
elderly, 38
electric blankets, 21
electrolyte imbalances, 135
electromagnetic fields, 15, 99
eliminative organs, 47
emotional conditions, 71
emotional reactions, 91, 95, 119
endocrine system effects, 18
endotoxins, 5
energy production, enhancing, 46
energy, assessing, 135
energy, focused, 17
enzymatic activity, normalizing, 14
Epstein-Barr virus, 41
estrogen, 82
exercise, 22, 57, 66
exotoxins, 5
exposure, reducing, 46
exudates, 14
eye conditions, 73
facial paralysis, 71
far infrared saunas, 28, 98
fasting, 22
fatigue, 118
   and liver toxicity, 83
fats and oils, 62
fever therapy, 21
fluoride, 4
food preparation, 64
foods, 61
four low electrolytes, 134
frame enclosure plans, 146
fungi, 13
gastroenteritis, 73
genetic effects, 18
genetics, improved, 14
Gerson, M., MD, vi, 89
guards for infrared lamps, 108

hair mineral analysis, 31, 120, 133
hair mineral laboratories, 136
headaches, 105
healing attitudes, 66
healing facilities, 51
healing reactions, 89, 118
   support, 94
   to slow down, 96
   versus disease reactions, 91
heat lamps. See infrared lamps
heat production, reduced, 12
heat shock proteins, 14, 23, 77, 85
heating the body, 42, 75
hemorrhoids, 73
high blood pressure, 36, 69
HIV, 69
home therapy, 51
hot and dry effects, 43
hot baths, 21
hot towels, 21
hot tubs, 21
hydrofluosilicic acid, 6
hyperestrinism, 82
hypertension, 36, 69
immune system effects, 18
immunity, 77
infections, 75, 94, 119
   acute, 78
   chronic, 79
   viral, 6
infections, mechanisms, 75
infectious disease, 75
infrared
   focused, 17
infrared benefits, 45
infrared energy, 97
infrared lamps, 109
   at the feet, 107
   at the head, 107
   breakage, 112

guards, 108
looking at, 113
safety, 112
why on one wall, 108
infrared light sauna
   benefits, 16
infrared light saunas, 28
   plans, 142
   problems, 113
insulation, 100
internal congestion, relieving, 12, 45
intestinal cancers, 73
intestinal infections, 19
ionizing radiation, 6
iron, 5, 121
Janov, A., 92
Jensen, B., ND, DC, vi, 89
jewelry, 37
joint pain, 149
Kelley, W.D., DDS, vi, 84
Kellogg, J.H., MD, vi, 2, 98
keloids, 72
kelp, 33, 121
Kervan, L., MD, 33
kidney effects, 18
Koch, W.F., MD, vi, 89
Kushi, M, vi
lamp safety, 112. See infrared lamps
lamps, infrared. See infrared lamps
layered toxins, 49
lead, 4, 121
leg ulcers, 72
light therapy, 77
lipid peroxidation, 16
liver, 82
liver effects, 18
liver toxicity, causes, 82
LSD, 36
lumbar strain, 72
lunches and dinners, 64
lupus, 73
lyme disease, 13, 75

166

mad cow disease, 25
magnesium, 121
manganese, 5, 25, 121
massage therapy, 57
meals, 39
medication, 37, 38, 67
menopausal symptoms, 73
menstruation, 37
mercury, 4
metabolic rate, 19
metallic pins, 37
migraine headaches, 105
milk, 62
mineral imbalances, 38
monitoring progress, 136
multiple chemical
    sensitivity, 70
multiple myeloma, 23
multiple sclerosis, 36, 73
muscle relaxation, 12
muscle spasms, 72
muscle strains, 149
musculo-skeletal
    conditions, 72
nerve root irritation, 71
nervous system disorders,
    71
nervous system effects, 18
neuritis, 71
neurodermatitis, 72
niacin, 58
nose bleeds, 72
nutrients, supplementary,
    65
odors, 119
organic chemicals, 105
osteoarthritis, 72
other therapies, 78
overdoing saunas, 39
oxygen production,
    enhancing, 16
oxygenation, 12, 45, 76
ozone, 58
Page, M., DDS, vi
pain, 27, 72, 95
pain relief, 16

pancreatic deficiency, 84
pancreatic enzymes, 84
pancreatitis, 73
parasites, 13, 73
parasympathetic
    dominance, 139
parasympathetic system,
    10, 137, 138
pelvic inflammation, 73
peripheral vessel dilation,
    12
pesticides, 3
pets, 39
pH balance, 86
pneumonia, 73
pores, unblocking, 19
portability, 102
positive mental attitude, 87
posture, 55
preferred minerals, 48
pregnancy, 37
prescription drugs, 83
Price, W., DDS, vi
prostheses, 37
protein, 61
psoriasis, 19, 72
psychedelic drugs, 36
radiant heating, 97
radioactive minerals, 13
rashes, 149
references, 157
reflexology, 57
renaturation of proteins, 24
replenishing minerals, 32
reproductive disorders, 73
respiratory conditions, 37
rest, 46, 66
rheumatoid arthritis, 72
ringing in the ears, 72
RNA transferase, 25
root canals, 88
salt, 32
sauna benefits, 10
sauna cabinets, 29
sauna research, 125
sauna sessions

before, 33
best times for, 30
body temperature, 32
cautions, 36
danger signals, 32
duration, 38
during and after, 34
how long, 31
how often, 31
supervision, 35
two phases, 9
sauna therapy
    how much, 32
    side effects/tolerance, 78
saunas
    and digestion, 77
    and spiritual
        development, 2
    body position, 105
    cabinets, 99
    cancer protocol, 87
    combining with other
        therapies, 78
    components, i
    convection, 97
    converting, 109
    cost, 30
    design, 97
    disclaimer, 141
    enclosures, 99
    far infrared, 28, 98
    frame, 110
    history, 2
    hot sand, 99
    in bathrooms and closets,
        111
    inability to heat up, 103
    infrared light, 28
    insulation, 100
    low-cost, 110
    materials, 100
    multiple person, 108
    odors, 119
    portability, 102
    power sources, 97
    radiant, 98

resources, 156
rotating inside, 113
seating position, 101
size, 100
solar, 99
traditional, 27
types, 27
ways to use, 2
scarring, 19
scars, 72
sciatica, 72
sea salt, 32
seating positions, 101
selenium, 5
sensory nerve damage, 39
silicone implants, 37
simple carbohydrates, 63
single infrared lamp
  benefits, 149
single lamp protocol, 149
sinus conditions, 72
skin, 19
skin activation, 42
skin conditions, 72
skin rashes, 119
smallpox, 80
sodium, 5
soft tissue injuries, 72

sore throats, 72
sound therapy, 54
spirituality, 2
spirochetes, 13
spleen and pancreas
  effects, 18
steam, 30, 57
steam baths, 21
stem cell, 81
sun damage, 72
sun poisoning, 19
supplements, 79
sweating, 11, 43
sweating, and infections,
  76
sympathetic dominance,
  135, 138
sympathetic inhibition, 44
  and detoxification, 47
sympathetic nervous
  system, 10, 137
  and cancer, 84
  and infections, 77
teeth, abscessed, 89
temperature, increased, 13
tendons and ligaments, 12
thermometers, 102
thermostats, 102

timers, 102
toxic chemicals, 3
toxic metals, 13. *See*
toxicity, assessing, 133
toxin elimination methods,
  46
toxins
  biological, 5
trophoblastic theory, 81
tumor necrosis, 87
ulcers, 19, 73
vaccines, 80
varicose veins, 73
vegetables, 62
ventilation, 103
vitamin D, 59
viruses, 13
water, 57, 64
  activation by infrared, 15
weight loss, 19
weight loss or gain, 96
wheat and spelt, 63
wheelchairs, 39
whiplash, 72
Wigmore, A, vi
yang effects, 43
yang therapy, 15, 17
zinc, 25